Prai:

The Acc....

"Melissa Jacobus' book, *The Accomplice*, asks us to confront the stigma and consequences of alcohol use during pregnancy. Though alcohol is a legally sold substance, blame and judgment against women and children affected by alcoholism run deep through the moral fabric of our society. This can be seen in the lack of awareness, even among physicians, of Fetal Alcohol Spectrum Disorders. What other disability would go so unaddressed and untreated over the past half-century despite affecting more children than autism, cerebral palsy, and Down Syndrome combined? *The Accomplice* is a call for us to provide diagnostic, treatment, and disability support services under the Individuals with Disabilities Act, which will help families like Melissa's feel less alone in their struggles to raise children to be independent and productive members of our society."

Douglas Waite, MD, FAAP
Chief, Developmental Pediatrics
BronxCare Health System

"An eloquent chronicle of a mother's endless struggle to raise two adopted children with Fetal Alcohol Spectrum Disorders (FASD), this poignant and moving book captivates and holds attention more than anything I have read about FASD in my many years of working as a forensic expert in the field. Lovingly and artfully crafted with the kind of insight into the disability no FASD 'expert'—clinical or forensic—could have unless they had raised a child with FASD, *The Accomplice* takes the reader on a riveting personal journey of what it is like to guide children through the challenge of transitioning into adulthood with a brain-based disability that is outwardly invisible but inwardly, mentally and behaviorally, disabling in a profound way. Simply put, every chapter is both instructive and a cliff-hanger. Readers will come away from reading this book as true 'experts' on FASD."

Natalie Novick Brown, PhD
Clinical and Forensic Psychologist
Assistant Clinical Professor (courtesy),
University of Washington, Seattle

"*The Accomplice* is a compelling story of a mother's heartache and her coming-of-age children struggling to find grown-up judgment to match their newfound spirit. Woven through her journey and the cause of her children's challenges are the bewildering effects of the most common yet most ignored developmental disability, Fetal Alcohol Spectrum Disorders. Overlooked or discounted by professionals and nearly every corner of society, parents are deemed to be at fault for their offspring's troubles, and affected children are labeled irredeemable. Melissa Jacobus shares a riveting saga of grief, ridicule, and hidden disability overcome by courage, love, and faith. Her story inspires the human spirit and issues a resounding call to prevent and heal a widespread disability too long ignored."

Tom Donaldson
President
National Organization on Fetal Alcohol Syndrome

"A heart-breaking, inspiring, and informative account of what it is like to raise or educate a child with a damaged brain caused by prenatal alcohol exposure. A must-read for anyone thinking of having or adopting a child, or struggling to help a child or adult who does not learn from experience and is a diagnostic puzzle. It also is a plea for society to understand the devastating nature of this very prevalent but largely unrecognized disorder, Fetal Alcohol Spectrum Disorders."

Stephen Greenspan, PhD
Emeritus Professor of Educational Psychology,
University of Connecticut
Author, *Anatomy of Foolishness*

"Melissa Jacobus writes from a mother's heart. Without realizing it, while she is pouring out her pain and sharing the hurtful and harmful struggles of her children, she is comforting others. She shares her story so that others will not feel alone on this very personal and difficult journey. Services and resources are greatly needed for FASD. Hopefully, this mother's love story for her children will reach an audience willing to educate and inform others to no longer willingly use alcohol prior to, or during, pregnancy."

Maggie Rousseau
Director of Disabilities Ministry
Office of Life, Dignity, and Justice
The Roman Catholic Archdiocese of Atlanta

The Accomplice

The Accomplice

Melissa Jacobus

BOOKLOGIX·
Alpharetta, GA

Some names and identifying details have been changed to protect the privacy of individuals.

The author has tried to recreate events, locations, and conversations from her memories of them. In some instances, in order to maintain their anonymity, the author has changed the names of individuals and places. She may also have changed some identifying characteristics and details such as physical attributes, occupations, and places of residence.

ISBN: 978-1-6653-0003-2 - Paperback
eISBN: 978-1-6653-0004-9 - ePub
eISBN: 978-1-6653-0005-6 - mobi

Library of Congress Control Number: 2021906884

Printed in the United States of America   040821

∞This paper meets the requirements of ANSI/NISO Z39.48-1992 (Permanence of Paper)

Cover Art by Evan L. Sykes

Mari Ann Stefanelli, Developmental and Line Editor
Kim Conrey, Editorial Assistant to the Author

The Accomplice *is dedicated to the memory of three people who inspired its writing:*

To Kim Lanier, a loving mother desperate to help her son, who she suspected was challenged with FASD. She was hopeful that one day she would find a diagnosis and the tools to help him.

To Dr. Carl Bell, a psychiatrist who called fetal alcohol exposure a crisis. His expertise and tireless FASD advocacy provided hope to all those who have been impacted by alcohol in utero. For his crusade for those with an FASD as published in his book, Fetal Alcohol Exposure in the African American Community. *And for his friendship and wisdom as he so eloquently expressed to me, "The truth is the light, so continue to have hope," as he encouraged my continued advocacy to bring the reality of FASD to the forefront.*

To my mother, Lillian Bick Jacobus, who passed away during the writing of this book, for her faith, prayers, and hope, knowing that the help of the Holy Spirit will never stop in this mission to advocate and bring greater FASD awareness to all those impacted.

Table of Contents

2015

Foreword

As we read *The Accomplice*, we were struck by three themes. First, Melissa Jacobus is a role-model mother and a highly experienced caregiver for people with FASD. Throughout this book, she eloquently points out that FASD is a lifelong condition. Second, children born with FASD are born with a developmental disability, and these neurobehavioral and neurodevelopmental deficits tend to get worse over time (Larry Burd and William Edwards, "Fetal Alcohol Spectrum Disorders: Implications for Attorneys and the Courts" [Chicago: American Bar Association (ABA), 2019]). Unless these children get the supportive services they need, they are unable to function independently. Early recognition and developmentally appropriate interventions are essential. Third, every child with FASD should receive services from their state department of developmental disabilities and receive special education services, mental health services, and individual therapies as needed. States such as Minnesota and Alaska include FASD or FAS as a developmental disability. However, in the state of Illinois diagnosable syndromes, such as Fetal Alcohol Syndrome, are not considered related conditions and do not qualify for services as a developmental disability. Georgia also does not recognize FASD as a developmental disability.

In the book *The Challenge of Fetal Alcohol Syndrome: Overcoming Secondary Disabilities*, the authors stress that secondary disabilities are problems that a person is not born with but might acquire as a result of having FASD, unrecognized FASD, or FASD misdiagnosed as something else (Mike Lowry and Michael Dorris, *The Challenge of Fetal Alcohol Syndrome: Overcoming Secondary Disabilities*, edited by Ann Streissguth and Jonathan Kanter, [Seattle, London: University of Washington Press, 1997]). These secondary disabilities include mental disorders, suicide attempts, drug and alcohol problems, anxiety disorders, post-traumatic stress disorders, inappropriate sexual behavior, and poor social and peer relationships. These conditions can be improved or even prevented with appropriate interventions and services. The book makes several recommendations about how states and the federal government can improve the lives of children and adults with FASD. One of those recommendations was for the United States government to change the federal definition of developmental disability to include FASD as one of the criteria for eligibility for receiving services. The authors also recommended that each state "develop and test modification of eligibility criteria for the division of developmental disabilities" to include FASD into their definition of what constitutes a developmental disability. People with FASD are often unable to live and work independently. They are often denied services when they have a full-scale IQ above 75. Despite having a higher IQ, one of the hallmark characteristics of FASD is having low adaptive behavioral skills. Having a diagnosis of FASD is equivalent of having an intellectual disability (Stephen Greenspan, Natalie Novick Brown, and William Edwards, "FASD and the Concept of 'Intellectual Disability Equivalence,'" in *Fetal Alcohol Spectrum Disorders in Adults: Ethical and Legal Perspectives*, edited by Monty Nelson and Marguerite Trussler [Amsterdam: Springer, 2015]).

In FASD, parenting is complex. We cannot underestimate how difficult it must be to know more about a problem affecting your children than almost anyone you will ever meet, including the professionals you reach out to for help. In Georgia, where Ms. Jacobus lives, and many other states, children in foster care are not routinely screened for FASD. Many school districts don't understand FASD and fail to provide the services needed for a child with FASD to get the necessary level of support for success.

Ms. Jacobus shares the reality of parenting children who have a brain-based disorder due to alcohol exposure in utero into their adult years.

This reality can begin with developmental delays and impulse control problems. This is often followed by unhelpful reassurance and incorrect suggestions that "better parenting" is the key to improvement. Parenting then devolves into a life of endless doctor visits and therapies (most of which have unproven effectiveness). This is followed by decades of trying to explain to people the unique needs of people with FASD: in foster care, at school, out of school, in the criminal justice system (including inmates on death row), in the employment world, in psychiatric hospital settings, to mental health providers, and in substance use disorder treatment. Then more explanations to your family and your friends. *This is the real face of FASD.* This is where diagnosis-informed intervention would be life-changing. A diagnosis of FASD predicts changes across the lifespan. A relevant example would be using the outcomes of assessment at age five to plan for the very different FASD-related problems experienced by sixteen-year-olds. The evaluation of school problems in elementary school has limited value for young adults in court. FASD changes across the life-span.

The most common misunderstanding among families, teachers, public defenders, prosecutors, judges, and mental health professionals is that the challenging behaviors seen among persons affected by FASD are a behavioral or psychiatric problem, rather than a neurological symptom of brain damage caused by prenatal alcohol exposure.

In the United States, Canada, Australia, and the United Kingdom, less than one percent of people with fetal alcohol spectrum disorder have been diagnosed. Diagnosis-informed care guides modifications of care to meet the individual person's needs. FASD is not an interchangeable diagnosis where FASD, ADHD, or substance abuse all mean the same thing. Intervention in FASD is different from other conditions. This makes a common disorder (12.5 million in these four countries above) a rare condition due to our inability to diagnose it. As a result, almost every person with FASD is destined to be diagnosed with, and treated for, something else. As researchers and clinicians, we can take some pride in our research population who nearly all have FASD, but we should also be very humbled by the 99.99 percent of people with FASD who are undiagnosed. (Svetlana Popova, Danijela Dozet, and Larry Burd, "Fetal Alcohol Spectrum Disorder: Can We Change the Future?" *Alcoholism: Clinical and Experimental Research* 44, no. 4 [2020]: 815-819, https://doi.org/10.1111/acer.14317).

As this book goes to print, we know that for every baby exposed to opiates, many more babies are exposed to alcohol. FASD is a more severe developmental disability, more prevalent than autism or ADHD, and more costly (Stephen Greenspan, Natalie Novick Brown, and William Edwards, "Determining Disability Severity Level for FASD: Assessing Extent of Impairment of Individuals and Conditions," in *FASD: A Guide for Forensic Mental Health Assessment*, edited by Natalie Novick Brown [Springer, in preparation 2020]).

This is the importance of this book. Ms. Jacobus is courageous to share her story—the story of the lived experience of FASD. She gives voice to so many families who, in quiet obscurity, are trying every day to make tomorrow better. It is clear now that the legacy of prenatal exposure to alcohol also impacts a large number of people associated with each person with FASD.

The Accomplice is a must-read for anyone who has been impacted by FASD. It is a textbook for training programs, and it is a call to action for federal government and state agencies that should be providing services. Most of all, it is a reminder to those of us who work with these families that we need to match their commitment—long days, sleepless nights, and weekends.

Diagnosis improves understanding and leads to services. It's now been nearly fifty years since the term fetal alcohol syndrome was identified by Kenneth Jones, MD, and David Smith, MD. Today, millions of people are affected by FASD (patients and families)—and they deserve better.

Dr. Larry Burd
Director, North Dakota Fetal Alcohol Syndrome Center
Professor, Department of Pediatrics,
University of North Dakota School of Medicine and Health Sciences
Justice Task Force, The National Organization on Fetal Alcohol Syndrome

William J. Edwards
Deputy Public Defender, Los Angeles County
Los Angeles County Mental Health Court
Board of Directors, The National Organization on Fetal Alcohol Syndrome
Chair, Justice Task Force, The National Organization on Fetal Alcohol
Syndrome

Author's Note

Years ago, when my children were in elementary school, their struggles with academics and unexplained behaviors, such as poor choices, understanding consequences, and difficulty with emotional regulation, were becoming more apparent. Teachers and pediatricians had limited answers.

As I searched further, a developmental-behavioral specialist told me that my children were most likely impacted by alcohol in utero. That specialist said I would never find the help my children needed in my lifetime, nor would my children receive help in their lifetime. I was advised to keep doing what I was doing to help them, but to realize their potential was limited because society was not educated on the dangers of alcohol in utero, nor the interventions needed for those impacted. The system was broken.

I was in disbelief, but now when I look back at that day, I'm also thankful. The specialist's prediction struck a nerve that threw me into advocacy. Advocacy that forever connects me with my children and others who are struggling with this invisible disability. As they are not invisible, they need hope and their lives deserve to have meaning. Our FASD advocacy is their lifeline.

The truth is, we've known the dangers of alcohol in utero for two thousand years. The Bible mentions this in Judges 13:7.

Despite that knowledge, the devastating effects of alcohol in utero continue today as those impacted try to navigate life with FASD. So it is with the story you're about to read. The challenges, courage, and hope for a better life are found within the pages of this book. I pray these words touch your heart, and if possible, please join the effort to fix this broken system.

2012

Chapter 1

It's Not Black or White

"Are you ready?" I called out to my son, Nicky, as I gathered materials to present at a seminar on the "invisible disability," Fetal Alcohol Spectrum Disorders, taking place later that morning. No one would ever suspect that Nicky was challenged with an FASD, a brain-based disorder attributed to his birth mother drinking alcohol while she was pregnant with him. The disorder is one hundred percent preventable; however, many women consume alcohol and don't realize they're pregnant, or they don't realize the devastating impact alcohol has on their unborn child. Boy, we had lots of work to do to educate people, which was the reason for the seminar.

I was proud of my son. Now twenty-one, Nicky had grown into a remarkable young man. In honor of his outstanding attitude and accomplishments, the state vocational rehabilitation department had honored him as a "Success Story" since participating in their program. In addition, the grocery store where he worked had recognized him as "Employee of the Month," and he'd received a "Shining Star" pin. Nicky is indeed a shining star to all who know him. Who would have ever thought he was capable of these accomplishments given his intellectual evaluations and testing results when he first arrived from the orphanage at the age of five? He was the cutest kid. Blond hair, fair skin, big blue eyes, and he needed to be wherever I thought he shouldn't be. Nicky was always interested in conversations; he seemed to understand but actually couldn't wrap his thoughts around the meaning. We jokingly called him the politician because of his talkative nature and charming ability to get what he wanted. School, however, was a massive struggle. Thankfully, the administrators of the Catholic school his three siblings attended understood Nicky's needs, and ours, which enabled all of our children to stay together. Nicky did countless hours of homework and was tutored just to keep up with his classmates. Weekends provided only a few hours of free time to simply hang out. He was the hardest-working "little man" I'd ever met. "Little man" was the nickname I'd given him to describe his determined work ethic and his thoughtful nature, which were far beyond his years.

When Nicky wasn't working on schoolwork, he took piano lessons, played cards, ping-pong, tennis, and anything outdoors that didn't involve multiple instructions and rules. He had great difficulty following along and frequently made up his own rules when he didn't grasp the ones others were following.

That didn't make him popular with the other students, which meant he had very few friends. Kids can be mean and Nicky felt their cruelty. Fortunately, one of the nicest boys in his class was also one of the most popular. He befriended Nicky, and it helped soften the bullying he experienced. We were forever thankful.

As we grabbed our materials for the presentation and rushed out the door, I found myself wondering if Nicky had brushed his teeth. This was a frequent reminder, whether he was five or twenty-one. When a child has an FASD, hygiene can be forgotten, but with repetition over time, it becomes more of a habit each day. It was exhausting to constantly repeat the obvious. For us, keeping a routine, being organized, providing structure, and emphasizing healthy habits made life easier. We didn't have to "think" about what came next. It became habit. We just went on autopilot, which made it much easier to get through the day.

Because today was FASD conference day, not Nicky's typical workday at the grocery store, the change in the schedule could throw the entire day into a tailspin of complications, forgetfulness into chaos, and frustration into emotional turbulence. Nicky knew the importance of raising awareness about this disability to a large group of people and the impact it could have for others who needed help. The attendees would be mostly social workers, psychologists, attorneys, teachers, counselors, and even those in the criminal justice system. Parents and caregivers would be present, though many rarely had time to attend a seminar as they were usually too busy providing care.

Perhaps there would be another person like Nicky, someone with an FASD, though it was unlikely. Those with an FASD might have difficulty focusing their attention and sitting for any length of time in a typical classroom setting, never mind in a room with two hundred people being instructed on this subject.

The seminar was taking place at the Georgia State Bar in Atlanta. For years, I had attended their seminar series, "Critical Issues Facing Special Needs and At-Risk Children." Many topics had been presented, but not FASD. This topic needed attention, as I believe it's the missing link to so many other co-occurring mental disorders, which are being addressed. But FASD was not well-known. It was not on the mental health radar, and I needed a carrot to get FASD into the seminar series. That had just happened in August when the American Bar Association had passed an FASD resolution, thanks in part to William Edwards, Deputy Public Defender III, Los Angeles County, California, Mental Health Court, along with other FASD experts. This resolution brought FASD awareness into the criminal justice system, educating attorneys about the possible mental health challenges of their clients so that they would be treated fairly. This was the carrot to get FASD on this year's schedule. When I contacted the Georgia State Bar about including FASD into this year's program, they said the schedule was full. Praying that a presenter would cancel and I could fill in with FASD, a month later I got the call. FASD was in.

The FASD presenters were varied, from researchers, psychologists, educators, and then me, a parent of children with an FASD. Although I was nervous, I knew sharing the day-to-day experience of caring for anyone with an FASD would shine a different light on this disability. Helping to organize and facilitate this presentation for the state bar was divine intervention. I was to speak in the afternoon session, and Nicky would distribute literature about FASD during the break periods. He had also agreed to answer any questions as he sat at the table with the various handout materials.

We got to the auditorium early to set up. Nicky was also nervous and concerned that someone might ask him a question he didn't understand. I suggested he give his usual honest answer of "I don't know." When someone with an FASD is put on the spot, "I don't know" is one of the most common responses. Nicky was comfortable with that answer, and I wasn't going to stress him out further. After we set up tables with the handouts, we were ready. A few of the other presenters came into the reception area and asked if Nicky could help them organize their materials on their tables. One of the FASD presenters, who had arrived late, had given Nicky so many instructions he began to shut down. This presenter was aware Nicky was impacted by an FASD, but she didn't understand his true difficulty. She gave him the instructions again, overloading him with more information. Frustrated, he looked at me for help. I told him to keep track of our material, and I would speak to her and not to worry.

She seemed to have limited understanding of the reality of how an FASD impacts the thinking of someone who is challenged, especially when that individual looks perfectly capable. Nicky's ability to communicate clearly, coupled with no physical signs of his disability, managed to fool even this doctor into thinking he could follow her multiple instructions. This "invisibility" is a trait of FASD. When a person with an FASD is overwhelmed, they often shut down in frustration because of their inability to process information. This can be confusing and looked upon as "willful" behavior. While it looks as if the person doesn't *want* to do something—it's that they *can't*. Although I tried to explain his challenges to her, she still had difficulty applying it to Nicky. At this point, I became frustrated with her inability to understand the disorder she would be presenting on. If a doctor has difficulty relating to it, how in the world is the public ever going to get it?

As the auditorium filled, attendees stopped at Nicky's table to look through the literature. I watched as some of them asked Nicky questions, and he handled those as he usually did, like a real pro. An FASD pro. And he was.

The presentations went well. A leading national public health institute provided an overview on FASD and presented on the statistical research. Other presenters focused on the impact of maternal substance abuse and the need to continue promoting preventive measures, stressing that no amount of alcohol is safe to drink while pregnant, and FASD is 100 percent preventable. The presenters used

PowerPoint slides, graphs, flow charts, and laser light pointers. All sophisticated technical tools.

Initially, the audience was engaged, but I noticed some seemed distracted by their laptops. Maybe I just had lots of experience homing in on inappropriate behaviors because raising my kids required lots of practice multi-tasking my peripheral vision, but it's amazing what I could see from the back of the auditorium. The audience was on social media or even online shopping. My kids have always said I picked up on other people's conversations, but this is one place I would have rather not been distracted.

As I sat there listening to the presenters, I noticed a young man in the middle of the auditorium, in the fifth row. He seemed to be about Nicky's age, and was obviously trying very hard to concentrate on the presentation. He fidgeted a bit in his seat, changing his position often. His eyes moved from one side of the room to the panel of presenters, then back down to the pamphlets in his hands. He didn't have a laptop, so I felt he was probably absorbing more information than other audience members. He stood out to me. It was apparent that he had more reason to be there than the few credits this seminar was offering—he was there to learn about his disability that no one understood.

The next presenter shared a wealth of information. She gave the clinical explanation for the different acronyms applied to the varying diagnoses from alcohol in utero: FAS (Fetal Alcohol Syndrome), pFAS (Partial FAS), and ARND (Alcohol-Related Neurodevelopmental Disorder). FASD, the "invisible disability," is an umbrella term that's used to describe the range of effects that can occur in an individual with prenatal alcohol exposure. These effects can have life-long implications, including physical, mental, behavior, and/or learning issues.

It was the end of the first half of the seminar and almost time to break for lunch. About fifteen minutes was left for Q&A. Those asking questions would raise their hands, the moderator would bring them the microphone to speak, and others would follow suit. The young man I'd noticed earlier, fidgeting though respectful, had been raising his hand for a bit of time. I thought how courageous he was to ask a question among this professional audience. When called upon, he said he was confused by the diagnosis he had received in the past in relation to what he was now hearing during the presentations. He asked the panel for help, looking for some clarity on what he should do. As he waited for a response, my heart was pounding and my hands were sweating with the nervousness he must have been feeling. The doctor who had just presented answered the young man, saying that he would need to go to a physician and talk about his specific personal issue.

That was it.

Not "see me after the presentation and I'll help you." How did this young man feel? How did he muster the strength to ask such a personal question, giving the entire audience a glimpse into his world? No one came to his defense, including me. We were all paralyzed.

We would break for lunch and return in an hour. I quickly got up from my seat, motioning to Nicky from across the room to meet me at the door. I was on a mission to find and possibly help the young man during our break, and if lucky enough, to have lunch with him. As Nicky and I left the room, we spotted the young man and a woman walking ahead of us. As we tried to catch up to them, Nicky and I discussed the response the doctor gave to this young man. Nicky commented that he wanted to cry when he heard it.

Catching up to them, we quickly introduced ourselves as we walked together. The young man reached out his right hand. With a firm handshake, he said, "Hi, I'm Maurice." He was as sweet and friendly as we expected. The woman with him leaned toward me and told me she was his foster care caseworker and worried about him. She filled me in about Maurice, saying he was twenty-one, aging out of foster care and planning on getting an apartment. She mentioned his challenges navigating life choices and trying to live on his own. She tried to convey as much as possible before they veered off in a different direction from the cafeteria.

It was heart-wrenching to think of Nicky, like Maurice, on his own, unable to properly care for himself. Nicky and Maurice were so similar. The boys were in harmony with each other, though the rest of the world couldn't fathom their struggles. Imagining Nicky homeless, which was bound to be Maurice's future, was unthinkable.

Nicky and I spoke about Maurice over lunch. We agreed about Maurice needing help, a home, and why not with us? We decided we would find Maurice and his caseworker at the end of the conference and exchange information.

As we returned to the FASD conference, it was my turn to present. I put up my one slide of me and my children. It was our "perfect family" Christmas picture. No one ever knew the struggles in our family. I wanted my children's lives to be happy, normal, and uncomplicated. My kids were okay—no pregnancies, drugs, alcohol, and certainly no arrests. I knew what the future could hold for a child challenged with an FASD. Their future, at this age, was like a ticking time bomb. As I discussed some of the personal challenges of having children with an FASD, I could see jaws drop and heads nodding. As I discussed the struggles of day-to-day life, the land mines in my own home, and the feeling of helplessness, not hopelessness, the attendees' emotions reflected my own. Navigating my children into adulthood was key, especially given the challenges of parenting hormonal teens in this digital world. These risk factors, coupled with FASD, could lead them into chaos.

As I continued speaking, my voice cracked. I couldn't look at the young man in the fifth row for fear I would burst into tears, knowing he was living through the same challenges my kids were experiencing, without the level of support I was able to provide to them. And who knows what he had already endured. Did he have someone telling him life was going to be okay? We try, try, and try some more? We never give up? Or that it was time to go to his grandmother's house to have Sunday dinner? It broke my heart. I knew so many of these kids don't have support and are blamed for their behavior and choices. They're told they're not trying, not understanding consequences, and not learning from their poor choices. Yet all the while, no one understands *why* they are challenged. The caregivers are faced with the same lack of understanding, no support, and a similar frustration and pure exhaustion. After I completed my presentation and the conference ended, I knew Nicky and I would talk to Maurice. We would offer him our friendship and our help.

We never got the chance.

Although we scrambled to find him and his caseworker after the conference, our paths didn't cross.

As we drove home, our focus was on Maurice. Who would help him? Where would he live? Would he end up on the streets? Nicky worried about Maurice, fearful of him being alone, and how we could find him. Maybe Nicky also understood how it felt to be Maurice and was acting as Maurice's inner voice. I told Nicky it would be okay. We would try, try, and try some more, and we would never give up trying to find him. Although it was painful to think about Maurice's reality, I was again thankful my kids were safe, no drugs or alcohol, no criminal behavior, and no runaways. The protective shields I'd created were in place, along with endless prayers that this would be enough to keep them safe from what could possibly be waiting for them on the streets.

2014

Chapter 2

The Runaway

My daughter had been gone for less than twenty-four hours, but it seemed like months. When Natalia left that evening, she was screaming at me to give back the smartphone she had used to stay connected to her boy-friend. I didn't know she had a boyfriend or a smartphone, though I had provided her with a basic phone.

We had dealt with the misuse of these devices previous-ly. Inappropriate pictures had been taken and calling cards had been stolen from the local grocery store. As a result, technological devices had to be monitored carefully.

In the past six months, I'd noticed Natalia's behavior had become belligerent, oppositional, and detached. She had also been acting erratically and had a very short atten-tion span. For example, Natalia knew how to cook, but late-ly, she didn't even know how to operate the oven.

Suspicious of what might be going on, I checked her bedroom closet. Hidden in her jacket pockets and shoes were ear buds and phones. Here was the problem—the negative effect of technology was probably contributing to Natalia's recent behavioral issues because technology can have a devastating effect on people with FASD. It's similar to people with a traumatic brain injury who are advised to eliminate or minimize their screen time on a computer, smartphone, television, video games, etc.

Natalia had been diagnosed with Oppositional Defiant Disorder (ODD), and I feared what she would do if I simply took the devices away from her. When she was a child, if something was taken away from her, at times, she'd go into an unregulated emotional outburst. She was an adult now, and her behavior was questionable to the point of possibly threatening. If she knew I had found her hiding place and taken her phones, there would be trouble. Keeping her safe was a priority, and I needed to buy some time. Because Natalia had a habit of unintentionally breaking things, I didn't think she would suspect me if her phones were broken. She wasn't home, and I needed to act quickly to disable the phones and place them back into their hiding places. I took the devices to my workshop in the basement, took them apart, and tried desperately to put them in disrepair.

Employing a flathead screwdriver, steel wool pad, and anything I could find that might alter the workings of the phone, the battery, wires, or circuit board, I was like a mother gone mad! Frantically scratching, scraping, and cutting wires, I tried not to damage the phone's exterior, which would give away my seemingly convoluted way of protecting my daughter. Praying that I had finally broken the circuitry board, I put the phones back together, but they still worked.

"God, please give me a break here," I mumbled. "Help me break these phones."

Usually I prayed for God to help me fix something, not break it. Good Lord, how my praying habits had changed. Well, it worked! Thank you, God! I quickly put the phones back in their hiding places.

In addition to the arsenal of contraband technological devices in Natalia's bedroom, she'd come close to losing her job at a yogurt shop, which was a short distance from our home. A few months earlier, her employer had alerted me when Natalia continued to access the internet on their computer system, despite her employer's warnings not to use it. Natalia had been online, unsupervised, and now she was taking lengthy breaks to meet with the twenty-four-year-old man she had found through the internet. She contacted him by using her "trusted" coworker's smartphone, then leaving the shop with this guy whose character was questionable, all while naïvely putting her coworkers at risk. They had been covering for her and now it was taking its toll. Her coworkers were frustrated with her and had alerted the employer.

Getting a call from my kid's employer was not the worst thing that could happen. This employer was sharp, kind, and cared about Natalia. In fact, Natalia had been working there since the yogurt shop opened. No one would have ever thought that Natalia would take advantage of her employer in such a sneaky, though brash, way.

As her employer and I pulled together our timeline of

Natalia's strange behaviors, it was obvious she had been pulling a fast one that had gone on for months, leading up to the current crisis.

To help her, we needed to know the boyfriend's name and his background. Looking into someone's personal history can be pretty tricky, but I felt there was no choice when my child was at risk.

After I learned his name, the next step was to contact his parents. I knew mustering the nerve to call them, asking about their son's behavior, and filling them in on the most recent events would be extremely difficult. Parents are protective of their kids, and I wasn't sure which way this conversation would turn. Still, it wasn't *if* I should contact them, but *when* and how will they respond? What did I have to lose? I made the call and the boyfriend's mother was initially confused, then alarmed, but acted responsibly. She soon realized that she and I were in the same frame of mind about helping our kids. She told me that her son was temporarily living at home. He'd been arrested for drugs and was on probation. His parents were giving him one last chance to clean up his act, or he would be kicked out of their house. I empathized with her situation and offered my support.

Natalia wasn't over her head, yet. There was still a chance for her. The boyfriend's mother asked that we keep her son and Natalia separated, as having them together would only mean trouble.

That evening, as Natalia tried to get the phone from me, we struggled. We were on the upstairs landing, and just as

I realized that things were getting out of hand, she leapt forward to grab the phone, pushing me against the stair railing, the steps just inches from my feet. She swung out at me and I caught her arm. I gave her the phone and told her she could not have any contact with her boyfriend while living in the house.

She called me a few choice names, packed a backpack with clothes, and left.

When I checked her room that evening, I found an arsenal of electronic devices, but no drugs.

Her brain had been hijacked by the devices that connected her to the dark side.

Disbelief and conflicting thoughts filled my mind. Surely she would walk only a few blocks and miss the safety of her home and comfort of her warm bed. Nope! Maybe she'd come home in tears, saying she knew I was only trying to protect her, and we'd work it out. Nope! Maybe she'd thank me for all I had done to get her through parochial school, special needs school, home school, and tech school, and she would profusely apologize for her abusive, bratty behavior and ask for my forgiveness, begging me to let her come back home. Nope, nope, and nope.

That didn't happen in the real world of raising kids with an FASD disability, so it wasn't going to happen with Natalia. She had limited self-awareness of her behavior and the consequences of her actions.

Her rock bottom was deep. Just how deep, she was about to find out.

Chapter 3

Reckless Spending

It was day two and I hadn't heard from her. Although I was unsure if she was with the boyfriend or someone else, I found some peace in the conversation I'd had with the boyfriend's mother. I knew she was stable, which gave me some reassurance that he had a bit of normalcy in his life. Oddly, I welcomed having a little quiet in the house, though the sleepless nights of worrying about Natalia were not.

In the days that followed, there were no calls from Natalia. I didn't have her new phone number to call her, and she didn't have to contact me for money because she had access to her checking account. Thankfully, she had agreed to put me on as the co-account holder since she had trouble managing money, a common challenge for people with FASD. Over the years I'd spent untold hours with bank tellers and managers, working together to clean up FASD-related financial messes. We were now on a first-name basis.

Because I didn't know where Natalia was, it would be reassuring if I knew the location of the ATMs she used, as that would give me an indication of her whereabouts. All the time I had spent teaching her how to use a bank account and instructing her on careful spending was now going to be put to good use. Could she make good financial decisions living on her own, possibly one day using her savings for an apartment, car, insurance, and basic needs? Well, welcome to my dream world. What the heck was I thinking? I knew better. There was no way she was going to remember what she had learned growing up. She did not yet have the ability to make adult decisions, and if she had had her way, she might have spent her entire savings in a candy store.

So, what kind of candy was she buying now?

Her life began spiraling downward. Natalia's employer, whom I had met with on several occasions, called me because she wasn't showing up for work. I received email alerts about the money she was withdrawing—$900 from various ATMs in less than a week was troublesome, especially given her boyfriend's drug usage. Her checking account was being depleted. Thank God her savings were in a custodial account, at my urging and Natalia's agreement, to keep it safe. She could not get to it and neither could anyone else, except me.

Concerned about possible overdrafts, I went to the bank, and the bank manager assured me that because Natalia had only ATM capabilities, there was nothing to be worried about. Her account would just go down to a zero balance. Although her safety was my top priority, I was also concerned about my co-account status negatively impacting my financial stability or Nicky's since I was also on his account. The bank manager assured me that the accounts wouldn't be affected. My bank accounts and good credit history were secure.

They advised keeping her account open to track her location, as I had been doing, reassuring me that her account was safe from criminal activity. I was relieved she was running out of money because I knew she wouldn't be able to live on her own without it. Was there a possibility she would come running home? Certainly she would call because she now understood the safety of home versus the danger of living on the street.

Nope!

Chapter 4

The Unexpected Visitor

About three weeks later, the doorbell rang. I looked out the window and saw Natalia standing on the doorstep.

She was dressed like a streetwalker, and a guy was with her. Was this her boyfriend? I couldn't get a good look at him and didn't see a large, luxury '70s Cadillac with a furry steering wheel parked on the street. It must be a boyfriend. Impatient, they banged on the door, yelling for us to come open it. Frightened, Nicky begged me to call the police as a precaution. At this point, I also felt police presence was a good idea and made the call.

Without waiting for officers to arrive, I opened the door. Still shocked, I was unable to speak to Natalia.

"Hello, Natalia's mom. We're here to get Natalia's money that is rightfully hers."

I didn't want to acknowledge him or his demands, and I responded with reluctance. "And who are you?" He seemed unable to process my question, so I added, "Are you Natalia's boyfriend from the yogurt shop?"

"No, he's bad news and on drugs. He was arrested. I won't let him around Natalia."

As he threw Natalia's boyfriend under the bus, it was obvious to me he was trying to come off as Natalia's knight in shining armor. And it was evident to me there was something very odd about his behavior. I knew I would have to manage him with care to get any information that would help Natalia.

"Good to know that you're not THAT boyfriend. What is your name?"

"His name is Max—" Natalia broke in, but he told her not to speak, and he was in control of the conversation.

"We want the money from her bank account. I have been in touch with a lawyer and will sue you to get it."

The nerve of this little flea standing on my doorstep, telling me to release the money that I had both helped and carefully coached Natalia to save over the years. I looked at Natalia and reminded her it would be available when she turned twenty-one, which was only a few months away. She could access the money then.

Max continued to threaten that he would sue me. His appearance, manner of speech, and limited eye contact were familiar, but I had never met him. He was talkative, rambling with little reasoning. Although he seemed somewhat intelligent, nothing he said made sense. Then I saw it—the invisible disability that influenced his behavior. Now that I understood, I began to feel empathy for him.

Still, I tried not to engage with him. His paranoia and oppositional behavior seemed to be triggered by his inability to reason or process information. He made no sense, but it was obvious he thought he did. He continued to tell me he needed access to Natalia's custodial account as she nodded in agreement.

I noticed she was wearing the simple, heirloom pearl necklace her grandmother had given her. Her grandmother was afraid she would pawn it for drugs. I told Natalia if she gave me the necklace, I would put money into her dwindling bank account. The gesture was also a way to pacify and ease them from the irate, unreasonable state they were in. Natalia gave me the necklace, and now I had to make good on my word. They seemed to calm down, a little.

Just then the police car pulled up to the house, and Max became agitated, saying that he'd done nothing to warrant the police. I explained that I initially thought he was the drug-addicted boyfriend, and I would talk to the police officer. After the officer got out of his car, I spoke with him privately, filling him in on Natalia's medical issues and recent behaviors along with the challenges at hand with Max. We thought it would be best if we spoke separately to the kids—divide and conquer. I would speak to Natalia and he would speak to Max.

Natalia told me she had met Max when he came into the yogurt shop. He was living on the street. She had continued the relationship via the internet and a phone she had received. Her information was vague, though there was enough about his family life that I could research and fill in the gaps at a later time. *Good Lord, more research. Here we go again.* Natalia revealed enough in our conversation that I suspected Max had been adopted, and his birth mother was an alcoholic. The traits of suspected FASD were being validated. I needed to learn more. Max's last name would be listed on the police report, which was public record, so I would have more information to go on. After the officer interviewed Max, he mentioned to me that he believed Max had mental challenges, perhaps bipolar disorder or something similar. I told him I believed Max could be challenged by an FASD, the same brain disorder as Natalia. As the saying goes, "Birds of a feather flock together," and Natalia had flown head-on into her nesting ground.

The police officer finished his report, with no charges filed. He cautioned the kids about their behavior, and I urged Natalia to come home and straighten out her life. She didn't agree. She and Max left the yard the way they had come, on foot, not driving off in a large, luxury Cadillac with a furry steering wheel and dice hanging from the rearview mirror. However, I didn't think this would be far-fetched in the future.

The police officer had handled the situation like a therapist. Careful, methodical, and calm, he'd asked questions to document the facts. I was relieved how well he worked with Max, in particular, as I believed Max might be a loose cannon. As the police officer questioned me further about Natalia's mental challenges, it was obvious he wasn't familiar with FASD, but he was interested in learning more. I would make sure he had his PhD in FASD after talking with me.

I explained FASD was similar to a traumatic brain injury, though caused by alcohol consumption in utero. Many of these kids become homeless adults and a high percentage end up in jail because of their poor judgment, risky behavior, limited understanding of the consequences of their actions, and suggestibility. The officer continued asking questions. I told him FASD manifests itself differently in each person, but with it being an "invisible disability," it was difficult to recognize. People with FASD can unintentionally fool others because despite the disability, they can appear credible, believable, and mature. People with FASD can have an average to high IQ, although they have adaptive behavior challenges. Adaptive behavior refers to everyday skills or tasks that the average person can complete. It reflects an individual's social and practical competence to meet the demands of everyday living with success. In other words, a person with FASD often has trouble managing the simple daily tasks required of an adult.

At that moment, Nicky, who had been silent but present during the entire "domestic" event, reached out and shook the officer's hand. He introduced himself as the one who was responsible for calling the police. "My mom takes on a lot, and she didn't need this, too."

Nicky was brave and protective of me. He showed great judgment in knowing the police needed to be called, and I was grateful that he had insisted.

The officer thanked Nicky and acknowledged his smart decision in this situation. He asked Nicky a few questions about what had happened. Nicky answered, stating only the facts, without any indication that he was frightened, just concerned about me. As Nicky's responses and factual account were incredibly mature, the officer had no idea that Nicky was also impacted by an FASD.

The officer thanked us again, reminding us to call 911 if anything else should happen. As he walked away, Nicky encouraged me to give the officer some FASD literature, as I never neglect a teaching moment. I ran inside to grab the easily accessible literature from my desk, then caught up to the officer as he was entering his car. I gave him the material and revealed that Nicky was also impacted by an FASD. The officer looked at me, puzzled, not realizing to what degree Nicky was challenged, or if I was a lunatic mom who thought everyone was impacted by an FASD. I had seen that look before and let it go.

I walked to the front door where Nicky was standing and apologized for having to prompt me to give the FASD literature to the officer. Ignoring my apology, he couldn't take his eyes from the police car. He was much more focused now than he was earlier. I realized Nicky's fascination with cars, especially fire trucks and police cars, was far more important than what his sister was up to. The police officer continued sitting in his car, perhaps finishing his report. Nicky leaned down to me and whispered. I knew he deserved this one request. As the police officer started his car, I motioned to him. When he acknowledged me, I asked if he would flash his lights as Nicky was eagerly waiting to see them. Curious, he then smiled and flashed his police lights. Nicky waved to him as he drove off. The police officer, waving back, understood.

Chapter 5

The Bargain Weekly Rate

I knew Natalia and Max would return when the money wasn't deposited into her bank account. As I was ruminating about my options for handling this, Nicky reminded me how I seem to always take on these responsibilities, and it was time for his dad to do something to help. When we adopted the children, we'd been married for twelve years and divorced six years later. Life with our new family had seemed normal, other than a transitional period due to a language barrier. Because the children had lived in an orphanage for some time, we thought they might have special needs. As time went on, the orphanage environment seemed less of an obstacle than their developmental challenges. As the saying goes, nature versus nurture, and it seemed that this was nature.

Disabilities were becoming more evident, though my husband wasn't addressing them the way I was. In addition to tutoring and reading to my children, I was focused on finding additional support, such as specialized tutors and Individual Education Plans (IEP). The truth is, children with FASD challenges can even fool their parents. Their expressive language, though it can be compromised, is better than their receptive language. So it becomes confusing when children acknowledge that they understand something with an "uh huh" and a nod, then can't follow through. To the untrained eye it looks like willful behavior. At times, they won't do what is supposed to be done no matter how many times they say they will, and they continue to nod or repeat your words that they understand what you're saying to them. Or so you think! Again, the adaptive behaviors can be compromised even though the IQ might be average to above average. It's a confusing disability that their father, my ex-husband, DS, didn't understand, along with many other unsuspecting caregivers and educators.

Nevertheless, right now I was in a bind with Natalia and Max, and I was desperate to keep Nicky safe. Reluctantly, I agreed that it might be time to call Natalia's dad, even against my better judgment. Big mistake!

I made the call, and when DS found out about the custodial account, he felt it should be turned over to him so that Natalia and Max would come to him for help and not show up at my house again, thus keeping Nicky safe. However, it wasn't Natalia and Max who raised my concern, but the potentially harmful people that they were connected to. With FASD, the challenges also tend to include poor judgment, lack of common sense, and naïve to the point of trusting dangerous people. People with FASD are gullible and vulnerable. I agreed to turn over the custodial account money, but only on the condition that we agreed upon—we would set up a police welfare check meeting with Natalia and Max and an intervention specialist to determine that drugs/alcohol were not involved. Then we would use the money to set her up in an apartment, safe and far from her current location. The money would be used for her living expenses, finding a job, and getting her on the right path. It would be interdependence, with the guidance of protective factors. He agreed.

Late that afternoon we met with Natalia and Max in a gas station parking lot.

"Hi Mom."

"Hi Natalia."

"Hi Pop. This is Max."

Max reached out to shake his hand.

DS rejected the handshake and said, "Why would I shake your hand? Leave my daughter alone."

What a mess! Max and DS were like two hungry pit bulls sinking their teeth into abusive words, which did nothing but escalate the already-tense situation. It was obvious neither was processing the other's words, and Max's body language made it apparent he wasn't processing the information. His frustration was mounting and explosive behavior might be inevitable. Max quickly removed himself from the fight with Natalia's dad to escape what he didn't understand. Seeing the opportunity to speak to them separately, I went to Max while DS had a chance to speak with Natalia without Max hovering.

"Natalia's mom, what about the money you promised?" Max said. "She gave you the necklace back."

Needing them to trust me, I made good on my word, and handed him the $20 I had in my wallet. I glanced at Natalia and her dad as they witnessed Max taking the money and leaving on foot.

Natalia, frustrated and appearing empathetic toward Max, looked at us and followed him, although he never spared a glance back to make sure she was there.

DS called to Natalia, "Natalia, are you kidding me? He's leaving you behind! Why would you even consider going with him? He only cares about himself!"

As the aching in the pit of my stomach intensified, I realized this situation had been handled horribly, and I was now questioning myself for agreeing to meet with them under these circumstances and releasing the custodial money.

The meeting with the intervention specialist, a "welfare check" on Natalia, was set up for the following day. I prayed that the specialist would already know about FASD, and I could get Natalia out of harm's way and this nightmare would be over.

The next evening, I met the intervention specialist and DS at a barbecue restaurant close to the hotel where Natalia and Max were staying, and we planned our strategy. Really, it was their strategy. They suggested I wait in the parking lot while they entered the hotel room with the police. I don't know what they were thinking they would find—drugs, alcohol? Some substance they think would have altered the kids' brains into this complex state? I knew it was FASD that altered their common sense and judgment.

The intervention specialist sat at the table researching Max's and Natalia's Facebook pages on her laptop. Max had multiple accounts, some filled with disturbing images. As they pointed out various posts that reflected his instability, I tried to explain FASD.

"Excuse me, are you aware of the challenges of FASD?"

Entrenched in what they were seeing on Max's pages, they did not look up or acknowledge what I was saying.

"Are you aware of FASD? Have you heard of it? Please look at the materials I've brought with me. Natalia is challenged with an FASD, and I believe Max is, too. If you understand this disability, you'll have a better grasp on how to help them."

Finally, the intervention specialist looked up.

"Will you please let me explain this to you?"

"Oh, yes, go ahead."

"Well, it's difficult with you looking at his Facebook page."

"No, it's not. I can multitask."

"Well, I can't, and I need you to listen and read this information. It will help you understand the situation you are about to walk into."

She then looked away from the Facebook page to listen.

After getting a crash course in FASD, they left the restaurant and went to the hotel where two officers were waiting. A short time later, they exited the hotel.

The officer said no drugs or alcohol were found, but added, "These kids seem to have some kind of mental disorder and are very immature. We can't arrest them or commit them."

The intervention specialist agreed with the officer's assessment, and I could see she was beginning to understand the perplexing nature of FASD.

DS informed me that he told Natalia he had the custodial funds, and she would have to contact him if she wanted them after she turned twenty-one.

The intervention was what I expected. Nothing happened except it validated the need to set up Natalia in an apartment away from this hotel, using the custodial money to manage her living situation. She wanted independence, not dependency. What she needed was an "environmental prescription," a term and concept I'd created that included a life coach, safe housing, support, protective factors, and interdependence. And that is what would happen on Saturday, as her dad and I agreed, if drugs and alcohol were not involved.

That evening, DS promised we would meet the next morning. I was to pack up Natalia's belongings from the house, he would bring the money, and we would get Natalia and set her up in an apartment.

The next morning, I had the car packed and was ready to meet Natalia's dad. I called several times, but there was no answer. When I finally reached DS, he said he could not meet because he was in a conference all day. We would meet on Monday.

On Monday, he had the same response. It was evident he had other plans.

On Wednesday, Natalia called me as she and Max were trying to find her dad to get the money he had promised her.

"Mom, Pop told me to call him, and he would give me the money. He's in Florida. Where's the money you said you'd put in my account and what about the necklace?"

"Natalia, let me see what I can do."

When I called him, he confirmed he was in Florida and that he wasn't planning on ever meeting to set Natalia up in an apartment with Max.

I called the intervention specialist, who told me to do what was needed. I would pay for a temporary stay at the hotel they were living in to keep them stable, make sure they had food, and return the necklace as I had promised. She strongly suggested that I get the custodial money returned to me.

When I called Natalia to tell her my plans, Max answered.

"Yes, this is Max, how can I help you?"

"Max, let me talk to Natalia."

"I'm so sorry, but you're going to have to go through me. I'm Natalia's protector now. Where's the money?"

I knew I needed to immediately change my tone of voice from authoritative to compassionate.

"Max, how are you both doing? It would be helpful if you put me on speakerphone so I can talk to both of you."

He did and I continued.

"Max, you sound like you might be catching a cold? I could tell when my kids were getting sick, just by smelling their face. Remember, Natalia?"

"That's right, Mom, you could."

"Yes, Ms. Jacobus, I'm not feeling that well. I do think I'm getting a cold."

"Well, Max, I hope you start feeling better. Get some rest and eat right."

Now, prayerfully, I hoped they would listen to me with no oppositional behavior. "I am going to pay for about five days for you both at the hotel until your dad returns."

Max quickly jumped in. "Oh, that's wonderful. But get the bargain weekly rate because it's cheaper than the five days. Thank you so much. Can you come and pick us up on the street? We're walking to your house."

"No, Max. I'm not at home and when you return to the hotel, the payment will have been made to the hotel."

"Okay, thank you very much."

I heard Natalia in the background.

"Thank you, Mom. Love you!"

It's like they were different kids.

As I scrambled to find my purse, I decided to return the necklace that Natalia had given me. She cherished the necklace, which had been given to her by her babushka, the Russian word for grandmother. Having that reminder of sentimental contact was important to her connection to stability and nurturing. I prayed she wouldn't pawn it!

When I arrived at the hotel I met with the front desk manager, who was guarded but sincere. I gave him money for a week's stay, an envelope with Natalia's necklace, and a gift card for groceries. He promised he would make sure it was secure until he could give it to Natalia and Max. I gave him my "FASD parent advocate" card, which made me an official wackadoodle parent trying to help her kid!

He told me that he had seen Natalia sitting in the lobby watching TV while Max was out during the day. They had been crashing in various hotel rooms. How they arranged it he had no idea, but together, we knew it wasn't a good situation. He said because Natalia was challenged with an impairment that disabled her moral and behavioral compass and her ability to make safe choices, he would act as an informant to help me and would keep in contact. Telling me I was a good parent, he also said he would keep her in prayer. How I needed to hear his support. My emotions came spilling out with no advanced warning, and I dried my eyes once more. *How could I seem strong when the tears were flowing?* I was relieved such a kind person was managing the hotel; he was like an angel in disguise. I thanked him and left.

The next day, for detective purposes, I set up a pseudo-Facebook page to track Natalia's whereabouts. Wondering why Natalia's dad was in Florida instead of helping Natalia as he had promised, I also searched for him. And there it was. The reason for him not being available for Natalia. He was in Florida at the beach. It was infuriating for me, and I could only imagine that it was infuriating for Natalia as well.

People who don't understand FASD don't understand the true crisis and what's needed for stability. Caregivers who don't have the support of someone who understands FASD know that it's extremely difficult to successfully navigate the path for the person who's impacted. Even though I was on my own, I was back in the driver's seat where I needed to be. I believe DS thought Natalia made a willful choice, rather than impulsive poor judgment, which is indicative of FASD. Unfortunately, his response is not unlike the response from others who are fooled by FASD behaviors.

But in my world as a parent-caregiver, and in the world of those like Natalia and Max, it can be catastrophic.

And was this where it was heading? A relaxing sandy beach would be nice for me, too, but at this point, I couldn't put my head in the sand and ignore the situation. Instead, I put my head on my pillow and tried to get some sleep.

Chapter 6

Risky Behavior

The phone woke me at midnight. I didn't recognize the number but answered anyway. It was Natalia. As I tried to ask her questions about her location, she hung up before I could get any concrete information. I looked up the number and found out it was a hotel in South Atlanta.

Over the next couple of days, I contacted the local police department and the hotel that Natalia had called from. When I finally reached the hotel clerk, I explained the situation. Although Natalia was twenty years old and no longer a minor, which makes it very difficult to get police assistance, the fact she has a neurobehavioral disorder called FASD compounds the situation. I let the clerk know that FASD manifests itself in many ways, including a possible delay in emotional age, intellectual deficits, and a limited understanding of reality that can lead to risky behavior. In Natalia's case, her poor judgment and impulsiveness can make it very difficult for her to make good choices. She was particularly vulnerable when she was around others with poor judgment, as she was likely to copy their behaviors.

While speaking with the hotel clerk, we realized the best

approach to finding Natalia was for me to go to the hotel and look through their security camera footage. Then I could copy any footage of Natalia onto a thumb drive. I began researching my computer's compatibility with their system.

For the love of God, I'm just a mom, and now I had to become an expert "IT" detective to locate her.

I decided I'd take some much-needed time for prayer, then leave for the hotel in the afternoon.

As I prayed for guidance, the phone rang. It was my friend Diane. When I told her the mission I was about to embark on, she insisted that she ride along. Diane is the kind of friend who has my back, no matter the circumstances. Even when neither of us knew what we would find on the other end.

The drive to south Atlanta seemed longer than the usual hour. Diane and I used the time to discuss various scenarios we might encounter. We were a little apprehensive, though not afraid. As we drove closer to the hotel, which was located in a high-crime area, we knew it wasn't like home and we didn't care. We would be one step closer to finding Natalia.

"There's nothing like a couple of badass women heading into a drug and sex trafficking area to find my daughter, is there?"

"And where are we going to find those badass women?" she said.

Laughing, I knew there was a reason she had come

along. We had just become "those women" and keeping our sense of humor intact would give us emotional ammunition. There was no turning back, knowing in just minutes we would be in the same area where Natalia had made the call. We were very aware of the danger that could meet us.

Driving up to the hotel, we scanned the area for danger. I pulled into the parking lot and backed into a parking space so my license plate wasn't visible. A black SUV pulled into the space next to me. The driver and passenger, two large men, looked our way. After a second glance, the driver rolled down his window. As the two men stared at my vehicle, I noticed they were wearing some type of police uniform, although their SUV was unmarked. Hesitant to talk to them and wondering if they were real police officers, I slowly rolled down my window. I took a big, deep breath and asked if they were from the local police department. I told them that I had tried to contact the police department over the weekend, and the office had been closed. Not missing a beat, they asked me what two women like us were doing at a hotel like this one. I refrained from a smart aleck answer.

They said they'd watched me pull off the interstate and followed my car, knowing it didn't belong in the area. They said they couldn't help but think of the line, "One of these things is not like the others," and wanted to know what kind of business we were doing. Their candid sense of humor was refreshing, and we proceeded to tell them we were looking for my daughter, a runaway who was hanging with the wrong crowd and had been at the hotel over the weekend. They instructed me to pull up to the front entrance of the hotel while they pulled in directly behind me.

Turns out they were indeed officers; in fact, they were members of the SWAT team and would be our hosts while we checked out the hotel. As we walked into the lobby, it was clear the hotel staff was familiar with the SWAT team. They all exchanged pleasantries as easily as they would with the mail carrier. Walking up to the counter, I wondered if the woman behind the desk was the person I had spoken to earlier. I hoped I wouldn't have to explain the situation again, as I had given her the information in detail.

"Hi, I'm Melissa and am looking for my daughter, who might have been here over the weekend. I spoke to a clerk who was very helpful on the phone." As she nodded her head, I knew she was the one I had spoken to.

"Yes, I remember speaking to you. The security system is not working properly, but I can get the footage if you can fix the machine."

With that, I walked behind the desk and kneeled on the floor where the security system was located. Thanks to my knowledge from a previous career, I knew to make a couple of adjustments to the equipment. It worked. Inserting my thumb drive, I began watching the footage, capturing the images of Natalia.

As I viewed the tapes for the next three hours, the two officers pointed out drug dealers and questionable characters entering and exiting the hotel as they also watched our backs. The hotel clerks, helpful though subtle, gave me information pertaining to my daughter and her arrival at the hotel. She and two other girls had come in through the back door late that Friday night, but they were accompanying the guy who checked in at the front lobby, paying for one night, single room. They were all in on it. Whatever "it" was. Natalia had carried the suitcases and various bags, which amused the clerks. This wasn't typical behavior for their regular customers. It was evident to them that she was in over her head.

Spotting Natalia on the security footage, my memories flooded back to the adoption agency's videotapes of her as a little girl at the orphanage, how precious, frail, and innocent she was. The two situations were so different, though I had many of the same feelings I'd had fifteen years earlier when I first laid my eyes on her—wondering how I would give her a sense of belonging and keep her protected.

I could tell from the hotel's security video that she wasn't aware of the danger she was in due to the choices she'd made. She flirted with the male hotel staff, which wouldn't have been tolerated by Max, had he seen it. Max seemed to be the ringleader of these three young women. As Natalia walked in and out of view of the security camera, it was more obvious that she wasn't aware of her own destructive behavior. The SWAT team officers cautioned me about the situation, as they didn't normally play host to detective moms trying to find their children. Though they understood, they reiterated their concern. Three hours later, I had what I needed. I knew my daughter was alive, the company she was keeping, and I had a copy of the footage I could use to find her.

As I lifted myself from the floor, dusting the cobwebs and other unknown substances from my clothes, I glanced over at Diane.

The older officer had taken her hand and placed something in it.

"Okay, sweetcakes, here's my card. If you or your friend need anything, call us. Now, since you got what you came for, you need to take your friend and go back where you came from. Where it's safe. We don't need to find you somewhere on these streets."

Hearing him instruct Diane with such concern, I realized we were playing a game of Russian roulette with this area, the hotel, and the people Natalia was running with. We were taking risks that could be catastrophic. She was in way over her head. And so were we. The SWAT team wouldn't be with us the next time . . . if there was a next time!

Chapter 7

Fraud

In a perfect world, we have enough time for everything we need to do. Time for appointments, time for family, time for work, and time for rest. For people with FASD, their time and schedules must be managed carefully, with structure and routine, because their disrupted schedules can impact everyone around them. When schedules are disrupted, it fosters mayhem and ignites stress.

Through the years of raising my kids, I learned to schedule important events early in the morning, as I never knew what I would encounter throughout the day. That habit still holds, and on this particular morning, I had an early appointment for a haircut, but needed to check my email first. When I did, I discovered that my bank account had been placed on hold. It was too early to call the bank, and I figured it might have been a glitch. I was confident it wasn't my banking error or Natalia's, as I had spoken to the bank manager after Natalia left home to make sure that her account was secure. The bank manager had told me to leave her account open as we might be able to locate her through the ATMs she used. Natalia could only withdraw money from her account, so there was no risk that she would be overdrawn. My account was sure to be fine. I had excellent credit and never had a problem. And if Natalia was out of money, certainly she would contact me. I would wait to hear from her.

Today was for me, at least for a few hours while I got my hair done. It would be a restful time with no thought of the chaos that consumed my days. Tony and Jackie, my hairstylists for over twenty years, knew about my kids and how stressful my life could be. They had that special nurturing gift of working their magic so I could forget about life's challenges for a few hours of "me" time. Though they would ask about the kids, they never judged. They listened if it was needed and gave advice if it was requested. The reality was that they always listened, and I always requested their advice. As the years went on, the challenges with my kids mounted. The "me" time was therapy, nonjudgmental and unconditional.

Upon leaving the salon, I checked my phone. There was a message from a woman named Karen, who said she had gotten my name off the internet from an FASD parent support list. Her voice was calm, though there was something about her delivery that seemed a bit panicked. I was familiar with calls like this and had left similar messages to other supportive parents or counselors back in the day. As the parent of children with FASD, I know when someone needs help, they're on borrowed time. They don't have much time to spend explaining the situation, and they try to fit it all in on a message for fear they won't have the opportunity another day. And then they pray for a return call.

Karen explained her situation. She and her husband had one child, adopted through foster care as an infant. At thirteen years of age he began showing signs of FASD. Though behavior typically becomes challenging with any teenager, these behaviors are more pronounced with FASD. He was now fifteen. She was worried because his disruptive behavior was not evident to others. God knows what she had endured for the past three years with his behaviors and her ability to keep it under the radar as "normal." Karen needed support. Ironically, she said she owned a salon and would need to call me in the evening. She said she had also sent me an email detailing her situation. I knew she was desperate and needed help because it's difficult to reach out to a stranger about parenting that seemingly isn't working. She was a caregiver, not just with her son, but to all those people coming into her salon for a few hours of "me" time. Now, she needed that "me" time, and I would make sure I was there for her.

When I arrived home that afternoon, I checked for the email from Karen. There was a glaring red alert from my bank. The bank account issue had not cleared up. It was not a problem with their website, but something or someone had suspended my accounts.

Since I had previously met with the bank branch manager concerning Natalia's account, I headed to the branch feeling confident I could clear up this mess. When I walked in, looking for the manager I had worked with for years, I discovered his office was now occupied by someone else. He had been transferred, so I met with the new branch manager and filled him in on the situation. He said $5,000 in fraudulent checks had been deposited into Natalia's account, and within a twenty-four-hour period, roughly $5,000 had been withdrawn from various ATMs. It was obvious this was professional criminal activity. The checks deposited into her account were preprinted, fraudulent checks from this bank and from a company in another state. They were made out to Natalia, but her name was misspelled, had the wrong home address, and the endorsement signature on the back of the check was not Natalia's. All of these safeguards had been completely ignored. To top it all off, her account had only forty-five cents left in it when the criminal activity took place. Certainly, the bank had better security measures than that!

I asked him how the bank could allow thieves to access my daughter's account under these circumstances. His response was unconscionable.

"Because you have good credit."

The bank manager would not allow me to access Natalia's account, my account, or Nicky's account as my name was on all three. Not only could I not access my money, the branch manager was insinuating I was the thief.

Thirty years with the same bank and I was being called a thief.

I was a victim of the bank's errors and the fraudulent check-writing criminals. Despite that, to gain access to my bank accounts, I needed to file a police report, contact the bank's fraud department, and prove my innocence. It was a catch-22. The whole time I'm thinking, *who's done this*, and *what has happened to Natalia?* Here I am, being called a criminal, desperate to find my daughter, and terrified of what the actual criminals might have done with my daughter. I knew that to have access to the bank's timeline of the ATM activity and to find Natalia, I'd have to follow the guidelines of this incompetent banking institution.

Once again, I was checking security videos, interviewing bank tellers, and doing detective work, due to the bank's substandard security measures. This required following the timeline to each compromised ATM machine. The bank's corporate fraud department mishandled the entire situation. All the preparation I'd done to protect Natalia from her own financial irresponsibility had actually opened the door to the thieves. I should have closed her account. The criminals evidently had one up on this banking establishment, and I was going to have one up on them also as I was determined to get the accounts open and remove my money from this reckless institution they called a bank.

That afternoon, in the bank manager's office, I was able to get information on one of the ATM locations that had been compromised so I could file a police report. After filing the police report and submitting the paperwork to their fraud department, my account was temporarily reopened while they conducted their investigation. If their investigation was anything like their inability to keep my account safe, I knew I would have to complete my own detective work. Finding Natalia, proving her innocence, and having money to access was not an easy feat. My day had just become a windstorm, and I was being blown in so many directions that it was almost impossible to stay sane in this tornado of insanity.

With the bank account temporarily reopened, I knew I had to remove my money and my son's money from this bank. I would have to leave Natalia's account alone. Fortunately, I had an established relationship with a particular bank clerk who, for years, had helped me navigate the accounts of my young adult children. I hoped the clerk would assist me with this transaction while the branch manager was out of the office. The clerk knew the sensitivity of the situation, was respected by the previous branch manager, and I went to him with my request for a cashier's check.

His subtle glance and acknowledgment of support for my family was all I needed to know he would help me as quickly as possible before the branch manager returned.

After the transaction was completed, now the question was where do I put my money? At this point, under my mattress seemed to be my best option!

In the past, it was extremely helpful to have our banking services in close proximity to our home. It encouraged some independence for my children, and it was easier for me to supervise this "independence," if needed. Those challenged with an FASD would like to be as independent as possible, but interdependence is the reality of a functioning life—support and a watchful eye from others abreast of the situation to act as their safety net when needed. This support needs to remain constant through their adult years as their challenges can cause conflict in managing their daily lives.

I knew I needed to focus on Natalia, her whereabouts, and the mess she was in, but I also needed to secure my family's personal and financial safety for Nicky.

The thieves had already found Natalia and her bank account information.

I wasn't going to let them get Nicky, too!

The Chase

A different banking institution had recently opened a few blocks from my home. Despite its reputation for high quality banking services, I must have looked like a deer in the headlights when I walked in and asked for the most experienced representative. It must have been obvious to them that something tragic had happened because three of their staff came to my aid. They brought me into an office, offered me a seat and something to drink. My first questions were, how secure would my money be and how much attention did they place on individual family situations? They didn't try to sell me on their packaged bank accounts, but were concerned for my family's well-being and listened as I briefed them on my situation with Natalia. They were shocked by the previous bank's treatment and assured me they would not have handled it the same way; they were even more concerned about my daughter's safety. We opened the new accounts, and they took every precaution to keep the money safe from further fraudulent activity.

As we were opening these new accounts, I discovered my previous banking establishment's fraud department had already put an alert on me. The cashier's check I had was good but my name was not. At this point, my new bank's personal banker knew my name needed to be cleared and directed the branch manager to set up a meeting with my previous bank that day. When he and I went to meet with them, the branch manager who had been no help to me earlier was conveniently unavailable. We met with another service representative, who said the banking institution would not clear my name unless I paid the $5,000 the criminals had taken due to the bank's own negligence. Disgusted with their lack of accountability, we left to regroup and strategize the next step.

That afternoon, my new personal banker, who was assisting me with the account, flagged the information and asked me a few questions about the branch manager at my former bank—the kind man who had assisted my family for years. The personal banker then excused himself from the room. A few minutes later, he had that branch manager on the phone along with the verbal and written authorization to clear my name of any wrongdoing. Then, after a quick lesson about Nicky's disability and why this mom was assisting her twenty-three-year-old adult son, my new banking team continued to set up my account as well as Nicky's, never missing a beat with understanding our family's banking needs, especially in this crisis. I knew we had found a family outside the confines of our home and in the most unlikely place, a bank. I knew from that meeting they would look after our personal well-being and would genuinely care about us. They knew I had to find my daughter and worrying about my bank account should not be my priority. Once again, I was free to play the part of detective mom to find Natalia, clear her name, and save her from the person, or persons, who were taking advantage of her disability for their gain.

Being trapped in an undiagnosed disability such as FASD is like being in a courtroom ready for judgment, but the jury has not heard any of the facts about the case. Nothing to go on, no witnesses coming forward in defense, not even the hope of a not guilty verdict because of extenuating circumstances. And the prisoner doesn't have the self-awareness to understand why no one is defending their case or the ability to defend themselves. The prisoner is frustrated, overwhelmed, and misunderstood.

It was going to be extremely difficult to prove Natalia's innocence unless I found the criminals who had taken advantage of her disability and vulnerability to pull her into their world of crime.

Now that my old bank had shut down my account, I no longer had access to its online records, including the ATM withdrawals. Fortunately, I had already filed the police report to open the criminal case with the bank, and that process had allowed me to access all my records before the bank closed my account permanently. Thank God I had saved and printed all this information. The first order of business was to review all the bank records, tracking each fraudulent ATM deposit and withdrawal.

Immediately I set out to get a detective on the case. I was willing to provide whatever information was needed to prove Natalia's innocence, but more importantly, I wanted to find her. She was obviously a victim, and I prayed the detective would try to protect Natalia and prove her innocence. That would be the easy part. Getting them to understand the underlying cause of her criminal act, the FASD, would be the hard part.

Navigating through the county's corrections system to find someone to help, I made countless calls and finally connected with a sergeant at the police department. He explained that check fraud is an everyday occurrence performed by what he called "recruiters." The recruiters enlist homeless, mentally disabled, or vulnerable victims who have active bank accounts. The recruiters manipulate their victims, taking their ATM cards with a promise to supply them with clothes, food, sleeping places, and a vehicle. In Natalia's case, they only took a portion to keep her trust. The sergeant told me that the force calls this type of case a "garbage" case. It's extremely hard to prove and make an arrest. The only reason he would pick up the case and assign it to a detective was because of my persistence.

Well, he didn't know how persistent I could be. I was annoyingly relentless and didn't care. I cared about Natalia.

I would provide them with all the information I had and would act like a sous chef or, better yet, sous detective! The sooner I sent them Natalia's medical history, along with

Natalia's fraudulent bank activity, the sooner I would get the videos released from the banking establishment's fraud department. The detective would act on Natalia's behalf, and I would back up what was needed, doing the work to get the information immediately. A detective was assigned and the process started!

In an organized and methodical manner, security camera footage from the ATM locations was requested and released from the banking establishment to the detective. The detective emailed the video to me, which I watched in the comfort of my home. The footage showed men making deposits and withdrawals using Natalia's ATM card at the different locations. Taking a closer look at the video, I noticed a cab was the getaway car. The same guys were in all the videos. Natalia was not in any of them. The last withdrawal from her account was at a branch in a nearby city, but video wasn't yet available. I called the bank and made an appointment to talk with the teller who handled the transaction. They could see me right away.

I threw on business attire, as I knew from previous experience that keeping myself looking stable, clean, and professional does matter when interrogating those who have information I need. If I came across as a lunatic, crazed, exhausted, desperate mom, they'd avoid me at all costs and probably throw me into the psych ward. Putting on the big "I'm doing great" front was a gift from God that I had honed over the years to help my kids, legally, at all costs.

I headed to the bank, which wasn't the branch I had

used in the past. In fact, I had never been to this location. I needed to speak with the teller and question them to see if Natalia had any involvement in the bank fraud. Walking into the branch, I signed in at the courtesy desk and took my seat. I wondered, *was this the way Natalia did it or was it even Natalia? Did she sign in and sit down or did she just go right up to the counter to get her money?* Scanning the room, I was looking for anyone who might have helped in the transaction that day. The bank manager guided me to her office, where I explained Natalia's disability and accompanying poor judgment and that recently someone had fraudulently used her account, which contained less than $10, yet $5,000 worth of fraudulent checks had been deposited within twenty-four hours and withdrawals were immediately made from an ATM. Certainly a teller would have picked up on this?

I had pictures of Natalia with me, though I wanted the teller to describe what Natalia looked like, in detail, before revealing her photo.

The teller who had handled the transaction joined us. He described the person making the transaction as a short, skinny, girl with long blonde hair, no glasses. He said she was dressed in Abercrombie & Fitch-style clothing. That would never happen with my budget! It couldn't have been Natalia. The only thing that could be remotely correct is that she is short!

When I showed him Natalia's picture, he said with confidence that Natalia was not the one who withdrew the money.

Relieved, I thanked them and left the branch.

The bigger question was, where was Natalia and who were the people in the video who took the money from her account?

I needed to email the detective and let her know Natalia hadn't made the withdrawal, and I hoped the detective would help me find Natalia and clear her name . . . so I thought. I was hopeful, but realistic, that the teller might have been wrong. For proof, I needed the video from the bank, and the detective was the only way I was going to retrieve it.

My hope was short-lived.

The detective's email was waiting for me when I got home. She had received the bank video, which showed Natalia making the transaction and receiving the money at the final location. They needed money and they got it, thinking it was legit. In the video, Max could be seen in the lobby, waiting for Natalia.

An arrest warrant would be filed.

Natalia hadn't just run away from home.

She was on the run!

Chapter 9

A Parent's Cry for Help

My daughter was a fugitive!

I pushed my anger aside and tried to understand her challenges. FASD is characterized by impulsivity, vulnerability, and a limited ability to understand consequences.

I could not allow myself the thought that she had been harmed and prayed that she wouldn't be. It would be too much to bear with the work I needed to do. In my heart, I knew she would be found. I also knew proving her innocence would be as challenging as proving her actions were due to her disability. It was hard enough to advocate for her throughout her elementary school years, never mind within the corrections system.

As I searched for information about prisoners impacted with FASD, the well was dry. Years earlier, I had been in touch with William Edwards, a public defender who works in the mental health courts in Los Angeles County, California. Billy is a highly respected attorney, an FASD expert, and was partly responsible for the American Bar Association's FASD resolution, which had been the catalyst for the FASD conference that I had co-led. *Would he remember me?*

But before I could find him on the internet, an email popped up from Karen, the woman who had left me a voicemail message earlier that day:

Hi,

I found your name on the national website. I have an adopted 15 yr old son and we recently have discovered his fas. I'm not handling it well. I don't know what to do for him. I am trying to get him in to drs. But they are months out. Can you please help?

Thanks,

Karen

I emailed her, and she responded that she was frustrated with his initial misdiagnosis and the lack of support she was receiving, yet she continued searching for ways to help him. Karen was in crisis and needed help. I emailed her with a possible time to talk. She responded immediately. She needed to talk, soon, later that evening if possible. Sensing her urgency, I agreed. We would talk that evening, after I'd pieced together the tangled mess that Natalia had gotten herself into, and I'd had a chance to catch my breath from the day's turmoil.

The call with Karen went longer than expected. Though she had educated herself on the clinical aspects of FASD, she needed the support and real-life experiences of someone parenting a child with an FASD. Her son, Jesse, was adopted as an infant through foster care. At that time, he had not been diagnosed with Fetal Alcohol Syndrome (FAS), which carries the criteria of specific, distinguishing facial features, which apparently Jesse did not present.

Jesse was now in his teens, and Karen was seeing unusual behaviors that suggested FASD. She didn't feel he was a physical threat, but he was lying, stealing, and had no accountability or ability to understand consequences. He had become more impulsive, with limited rational thinking.

Karen had just entered the world I'd been living in for the past ten years.

She told me that Jesse had been diagnosed with various developmental and intellectual disabilities, but she believed FASD had gone under the radar. Karen was smart and she was right on target. She was trying to educate the educators, doctors, and counselors about her experience with her son. I encouraged her to keep any therapist appointments she had, and I would send her FASD information to further educate those who didn't understand the disorder.

I explained that keeping Jesse mentally *under*-stimulated was a critical step to keep his brain rested. During the hormonal teen years, this can be particularly challenging due to the person's inability to regulate their emotions, overstimulation of screen time, and the unsupervised exposure to internet content. In other words, limit texting, gaming, and the influence of violent programming. The digital world can wreak havoc on people with FASD—the content children watch, how it's delivered through their thought processes, and the mental exhaustion it causes. I knew this all too well, and at those times, mental rest or physical activity was a lifesaver.

Karen got it! We spoke late into the night. We cried and we connected from the support we gave each other. I validated her suspicions that she needed help for her son, and she validated my thoughts that so many families out there were suffering and not getting the help they needed.

She was smart, strong, a loving caregiver, and deserved all the "me time" that she continued to give others in her life. We ended the call, and I emailed her the information I had promised, along with a message telling her she was a great mom, take heed of the cautionary red flags to stay safe, and she was going to be fine.

My faith and nightly prayers were important, though I was so tired this evening. Before I went to sleep, I prayed for Karen, her family, and those who would need to assist her. And as always, I prayed for Natalia's safe return and Nicky's continued stability. God help them all understand!

God help us all.

That was about the best I could do before falling asleep.

Chapter 10

Caring for Caregivers

Rest for a parent or caregiver of a child challenged with FASD is rare. It seems every waking moment, when not addressing the needs of your kids, you are defending yourself in how you parent them. If you're not stepping over emotional land mines or taking cover from chaos grenades, you're covering their backs from others' misconceptions about their behaviors and still having to cover your own back. If you don't, something is bound to sneak by you, which is difficult to recover from. FASD caregivers need respite, support, and a closet big enough to escape to when the world seems to be turning their backs on what you know to be obvious. You are judged for being too protective, then judged for not being protective enough. Those on the outside only experience the normalcy of your family but don't realize the extreme "environmental prescription" work needed to make everything look normal.

I remember one situation when my kids were in elementary school, and Nicky told the teacher he didn't get to eat dinner. I got a call from the principal that evening, looking for an explanation. Fortunately, she was an excellent school administrator and she knew one of our favorite teachers had made the report, and that teacher was looking out for her student. The principal also knew my history, that my children were adopted from orphanages. The confusion arose because my son had only told a portion of the story to the teacher. He's believable, and she lacked experience and knowledge about FASD. My son could be unintentionally convincing in a "woe-is-me" situation, all while radiating charm. He wasn't starved or chained to a bed post with mere crumbs and a drop of water to drink.

Here's the real story: In the evening, if any of the children were cranky, weren't getting along with other family members or misbehaving, they ate dinner earlier than everyone else and would go to bed early. Dinner would usually be plain oatmeal or flavored with blueberry or apples and cinnamon.

Heck, when I got in trouble as a kid, I went to bed without dinner. I was lucky if I got toothpaste to brush my teeth, which I loaded up on, thinking it would fill me up before my next meal in the morning.

As the principal listened to my explanation, she realized what my son had omitted from the conversation, which probably should have gone something like, "I don't get to eat dinner with the family when I'm misbehaving, but have to go to bed early after I eat my oatmeal." This lack of information can be misconstrued and shine a really bad light on parents or caregivers. I knew if this situation was any indication of what I had to look forward to during the teenage years, I'd better hone my tough-skinned parenting skills. As the saying goes: little kids, little problems; big kids, big problems. Who would have imagined some of what I was about to embark upon?

Throughout the elementary school years and into high school, school choices are limited when your children begin to show signs of special needs. Psych evaluations are lengthy, expensive, and not always right on point. FASD is still not understood as a known disability, and fifteen years ago when my children were young, no one understood these challenges or needs. I attended multiple conferences, gathered information for Individual Education Plans (IEPs), and tried to teach the school staff about the test results that they themselves misunderstood. One administrator, who had experience with children adopted from Russia, told me my children were bound to turn on me. Sadly, with what I was experiencing, I understood his comment. But the issue isn't ethnicity. Children who grow up to be adults with FASD are misunderstood. At one point, a neuropsychologist told me I was doing a great job parenting, but he suggested keeping the alcohol-induced brain disorder private. He felt the kids or my family would be ostracized or stigmatized.

I realized he could be right as I had already experienced this treatment, so I had to use care when addressing each audience. Depending on the situation and how it was perceived, teachers, other parents, doctors, friends, and even some relatives just didn't get it. They didn't *see* it. This is why FASD is called the "invisible disability." And many times I wanted to make myself invisible, as it is isolating. I want to run away from it. But I'm not going to. Withstanding the stigma and isolation is essential so that one day FASD will be understood by everyone as a brain-based developmental disability, and those impacted will have the opportunity for happy, productive lives. My children had gifts and strengths. They could navigate and overcome these challenges as they developed, if they had the right support, protective factors, and interventions to help them.

I was thankful for those who understood or at least tried. I was also thankful that I had my faith, which I leaned on heavily. You would think that God's shoulders were the size of Mount Rushmore, as much as I leaned on them. He was steadfast, patient, and nonjudgmental. I had many prayer talks with Him in that closet, asking for His guidance. In those moments of isolation, He was the rock that I rested on to keep our family together. Prayer and traditions were constant, which were probably what enabled us to avoid the sinkhole that could have swallowed up our family years earlier.

God help the caregivers and handle them with care!

Chapter 11

Homeless in DC

And that's what I wanted, for God to handle me with care. I was exhausted, overwhelmed, and just once I wanted someone else to step in and handle this constant deluge of chaos. But I needed to stay positive, so I ended my pity party and set out to find Natalia.

Where was she now? I had paid for only a week at the hotel and had not heard from her since. She'd been gone for three months. *Who had compromised her bank account? Was she alive and okay or curled up somewhere in the fetal position, scared and hungry? As she was so susceptible to others' influence, had she become part of their criminal behavior?* I got a cup of coffee and I headed upstairs to her bedroom. As I thought of Natalia and tried to put myself in her mindset, I realized she probably was unaware of the problems she had created for herself. With her limited self-awareness and impulsive nature, she lacked the ability to get out of the trouble she had "chosen."

I sipped on my coffee, analyzing the situation, and wandered around her bedroom. It was decorated in a horse motif, with many items she had collected through the years. Her room was filled with antiques we had found together, refinished together, and created a stable environment, her sanctuary of calm. One particular antique store we visited on Fridays after homeschooling was owned by a woman who connected with Natalia due to their shared love for horses, creativity with antiques, and ability to connect to the human spirit. Their connection was the inspiration for Natalia's room. I realized this woman was one of those angels who would re-enter our lives one day.

Natalia attended horse camp as a youngster, and the handler had mentioned many times that Natalia had a gift for connecting with these animals, beyond even some trainers. Even at such a young age it was evident to the handler that Natalia had an understanding, a trust, an unspoken language with horses. It seemed every time she came back from riding, her brain worked better. I found out in later years that the movement of riding horseback increases cognitive ability and stimulates a healthy brain. If only I could have continued to accommodate her needs in this way.

I refilled my cup before heading to my office in the basement. I wanted to get on my computer to try to put the pieces of the ATM scam together, and I began dissecting the bank statements and noting the ATM locations that were compromised the night of the fraudulent activity. I needed to find the ringleader of this crime. Here I was, playing detective, with a whole lot of emotion attached, in the hopes of locating Natalia.

As I began searching areas where she might be living, I thought of Maurice, the young man who had sought help at the FASD conference and was told to find a physician for a diagnosis. Was he wandering the streets, trying to find a place to call home or had he fallen victim to criminals taking advantage of him? People can easily take advantage of individuals with FASD because they're vulnerable to peer pressure. In addition to the challenges of understanding the consequences for their behavior, they often lack self-regulation and impulse control. My heart went out to Maurice.

The phone rang and I didn't recognize the number. *Could it be Natalia?*

"Hello?"

"May I speak to Melissa Jacobus?"

"Yes, this is Melissa."

"This is Agatha from a woman's homeless shelter in Washington, DC. We found your daughter Natalia, and for us to help we need her identification papers."

"Excuse me, who is this and where are you from? You're with Natalia?"

"My name is Agatha. I'm with a homeless outreach program. We found Natalia on the street, wandering in a daze."

Natalia had a history of appearing to be in a daze, but doctors had told us she might actually be having small seizures and to keep an eye on her. Well, that's all it took. I knew the outreach program had Natalia with them and she was now off the street. Keeping Agatha on the phone, I began to search for her on the internet, making sure her credentials were as she stated. She asked for specific identification papers: birth certificate, passport, and a doctor's diagnosis for Natalia to receive any mental health or welfare services. I was hesitant to give her the information until I confirmed she was who she said she was. In the wrong hands, this information could lead to more trouble with another scam. Though Natalia had given Agatha my name and phone number, Agatha wouldn't let me speak to her.

I mentioned Natalia has the "invisible disability" of FASD. Agatha had never heard of it.

She was very private with what she would reveal, and I knew I was going to have to play detective once more to look into Agatha's psyche. Although I dreaded Google and Facebook searches, they would help me find out why she wouldn't reveal more. It's amazing what people place on these transparent, social networking sites for the world to read.

Reading Agatha's Facebook page, it became apparent that she had preconceived ideas about the parents of the kids she found on the street. She was demonizing them as "parents who don't understand their kids and bad parenting" and stating that she understood these kids better than they did. I looked further into her posts and discovered she was having fertility problems and was seeking donations to help with medical expenses. If I related to her on this level, perhaps she would trust me enough to give me information about Natalia. I called her the next day and subtly mentioned I had not been able to get pregnant. Although I was an adoptive parent, it didn't change the love a mother has for her daughter. One doesn't have to be related by birth to connect to their children. Agatha and I connected, and she revealed more of what I needed to know.

She told me they had found Natalia on the street, wearing revealing clothing and acting in a dreamy, spacey manner. She was alone when they found her, though they met up with Max later. Both Natalia and Max were in their care at two different facilities. Agatha needed Natalia's identification papers to assist her in the women's shelter and expedite housing and mental health services. Once they got the information they needed, they would return it to me.

I sent the papers immediately, along with information about FASD, to arrive overnight. I finally got a restful night's sleep knowing that Natalia was alive and in the care of a medical facility where they could help her. Fearful it might disrupt the mental health assistance she would receive, I didn't mention a warrant for her arrest was going to be filed in Georgia.

For the next couple of days, which then became weeks, I called, sent emails, and received no response from Agatha. Concerned that Natalia was no longer there, I contacted a close friend who lived in DC. Mary Anne had known Natalia since the day she arrived from the orphanage. Mary Anne, sharp, capable, and caring, jumped at the chance to help.

She was one of God's angels, and on this occasion, Mary Anne visited the homeless facility and was told that Natalia was there, but she wasn't allowed to see her because of privacy laws. Mary Anne left a note and a phone number with the shelter to give to Natalia.

Still, there was no word from Agatha about Natalia, and it was time to go further up the chain of command to get some answers. It had been almost three weeks since Natalia was brought in from the street, but her whereabouts were still uncertain. Also, her ID papers had not been returned to me, as Agatha had promised. Emails and phone calls continued as I tried to find Natalia.

When I finally talked with Agatha about the ID papers, she said she had tried to send them, but she admitted she'd weighed the package on her kitchen cooking scale. The package had been returned for inadequate postage.

I had a sick pain in my stomach that something was horribly wrong. It had been a gnawing feeling since the day after Agatha had called to notify me that they had found her. A mother's instinct! I called the director of the facility, and she confirmed what I had feared.

Natalia left the facility the day after she arrived.

Finding trouble, again.

Chapter 12

Prince George's, She's in the Can

It didn't take long for Natalia and her boyfriend, Max, to explore the streets of DC. I didn't know where she was, and the shelter's director didn't have that information. That was for me to find out.

Completely exhausted by the past couple of months and sleepless nights, my mind was racing, wondering what steps I needed to take next. I searched for Natalia's name in various counties throughout DC and the surrounding areas. Retrieving inmate listings from jails was all new to me, thank God; I juggled between phone calls and frantically looking up information on my computer. I'd found Max's dad through the internet and left a message for him to contact me.

Max and Natalia had told me his parents had adopted him when he was a young teen. Many of his challenges were indicative of FASD.

My phone rang.

"Hello, this is Melissa."

"Hello, this is Max's dad. I got your message about Natalia."

I thanked him for calling me and said, "The kids are in trouble, and I believe Natalia is in jail. Have you heard from Max lately?"

"Yes, Max has been contacting me, and Natalia called me a few weeks ago. She was looking for Max so he could hire a lawyer to get her out of jail."

"You realize these kids have no idea what they are talking about or doing. How did they get in jail?"

"Apparently, they went off in a car with some guys to a park, and the guys had drugs in the car. Max and Natalia were not part of the drugs, but they were present when the driver was pulled over by the police. Max wasn't held, as it was a minor offense, but Natalia was. Why would they hold her?"

I proceeded to tell him about the whole ATM mess, the check fraud, and the hell I'd been living through, trying to clear the bank accounts and find Natalia. I also explained Natalia's history of FASD. Max's father had never heard of FASD, but said its characteristics seemed very similar to what he had experienced with Max. Max's dad told me they'd dealt with Max's behavior challenges, disrupted school experiences, and the many questionable diagnoses that he'd had over the years of living within the foster care system.

"What number did she call you from?"

"I'll have to hang up and check my phone."

"Okay, please call me right back."

As soon as he called me with the number, I searched the

internet for its location. The area code was Prince George's County, Maryland. All I could think of was the old-school pipe tobacco, Prince Albert, that was packaged in a tin or can, jokingly referred to as "Prince Albert in the can." And now it was Prince George's, and Natalia's in the can! Here I am, dealing with pure exhaustion and my mental state racing, and this was where my mind was going? Perhaps humor was a healthy distraction, lightening the severity of Natalia's situation so I wouldn't go crazy myself.

"She's in Prince George's in a can—I mean Prince George's County. When did she call you?"

"Sorry, let me look at it on my phone again and I'll call you right back."

It was obvious I was the one who had played detective all summer and honed my Columbo skills.

He called again. "Okay, I got it. She called September 24."

As we were talking, he had another call. He said it looked like a local call. I looked up the number as he rattled it off to me. It was a county in Georgia, close to home.

Natalia must have been extradited to Georgia. He was not going to accept the call, and I would wait to hear from her. I hung up and quickly called my friend Anita who had experience with the county jail as her teenaged children had challenges with FASD and the law. She explained that Natalia would be in a twenty-four-hour holding cell upon arrival and would be able to make a phone call to post bail. Anita gave me a quick rundown on what to expect and how I could assist her.

I would wait.

That afternoon, I got an email from the women's homeless shelter, saying Natalia was incarcerated in Maryland in September. Finally, they had come through with information, though too late.

Taking a moment to catch my breath and slow my heart rate, I found the documentation of Natalia's arrest on the internet.

She was listed as a FUGITIVE.

The phone rang.

"Hello?"

"Mom, this is Natalia. I'm in jail. I'm so sorry. I need help."

Relieved to hear her voice, I took a breath.

"I know . . . You'll get through this, Natalia. I'm here for you. A public defender will be assigned to you. Try to remember all that has happened and tell your public defender the truth."

"I don't remember, Mom. I have to go. I'll call you back tomorrow."

I could hear her crying as she said goodbye.

As the call ended, my heart sank. But she was safe, and I was thankful. I prayed that she would now understand the help that was available to her, and she would come to her senses and accept the help she needed. Or would she?

When she and I were talking, another call had come in on my phone. It was early evening and I was exhausted. Maybe I'd listen to the voice message tomorrow, rested and with a clear head. Certainly, the call could wait. What else could possibly happen? Taking a deep breath, I decided to listen to the message.

"Melissa, this is John, Karen's husband. When you get this message, will you please give me a call?" He left his number. "Thank you."

His voice was sweet, Southern, and frail. I recognized the name, Karen, and remembered speaking with her a month or so earlier. She was bright, a concerned mother, and I knew she would do whatever she could to help her son. She was one of those angels who had adopted a challenged child and taken him under her care to love and nurture, unselfishly.

When I returned her husband's call that evening, I never expected what I was about to hear.

Chapter 13

Dying for a Diagnosis

I flipped through the pages of the logbook where I kept my handwritten notes about the people who'd contacted me about FASD over the years. There were many pages and many calls. These caregivers, mostly parents, were brave to call, scared, frantic, and needing help. Spending time with them on the phone, sharing experiences, sending them resources, listening intently to their needs, and trying to assist them with the crisis at hand, all this was detailed on those pages. Sometimes I heard from them again, sometimes not.

I found that by the time a parent or caregiver, desperate for help, reaches out to an "expert" stranger, they have already exhausted all possible means of trial and error as they know it. Not only have they probably been through countless crisis situations, but they've felt hopeless. Many times, no one sees the behavioral and emotional challenges other than the caregiver or parent, who sees it twenty-four hours a day. And why aren't the professionals able to understand their child's situation? Then the parent-caregiver may have family members and friends that, unknowingly, may not be as supportive as they could be, again, because these family members and friends aren't seeing the behaviors. I know these caregivers have to be more than a helicopter parent; they have to be a strategic, military helicopter parent just to make life seem normal to the outside world. Then, as the child ages, the situation begins to take a downturn. Just as I did, the parents and caregivers will have to scramble just to keep their heads above water, gasping for air, as they throw a life raft to their child, who is ripping off their life jacket, in this massive whirlpool of FASD and no rescue in sight.

Checking my logbook, I read the notes I had taken when I talked with Karen a few months back. She was calm, stable, but scared of the behaviors she was beginning to see in Jesse, her fifteen-year-old son. Fortunately, she said she didn't feel physically threatened. Friends and family members were beginning to see her son's behavior challenges but passed them off as "almost normal" teenage behavior.

And that's the clincher. As a parent of an FASD child, they know it's more than "almost normal." They're not being an alarmist and know they need to take action. However, they are being judged as being overprotective and overconcerned. Then, when the odd behaviors start affecting others, they begin to further isolate themselves, trying to get a handle on the behaviors, which they know are not normal.

Karen got it. After doing her research, she was sure Jesse was challenged with an FASD. Her son was on a waiting list at an FAS clinic in Atlanta. She fully understood what she was about to encounter on the FASD path. She needed resources to support her intuition and experiences, which is what I provided, along with my support as a mother who has walked a similar path.

I warned her about the overstimulating effects of digital devices, and she said his were limited. They did watch family movies for entertainment. There was nothing wrong with this, though at his age anything even slightly violent or quick-cutting video was cautioned against. They didn't have video games in their home, and from what they knew, he had no exposure to them elsewhere.

Karen was sharp and heeded the warning. Most importantly, she loved her son and would do what she needed to keep him safe and educate others about his needs. She would continue to "keep herself safe" while advocating for him.

Her warm personality jumped off the pages of my notebook, and I knew she was a friend for life. We would meet again one day. So why was her husband calling me?

I dialed his number and he answered.

"Hello?"

"Hello, I'm returning a call from this afternoon. This is Melissa Jacobus."

"Hi, Melissa. Thank you for calling me back."

"You are so welcome. I recall talking with Karen several months ago when she called me about your son. She was concerned about recent behaviors and believed he might possibly be impacted by FASD."

"Yes, Melissa. She was so happy when she got off the phone with you. She said someone finally understood what we were experiencing with our son."

I remembered how Karen had cried in frustration from the isolation she felt and from the professionals that dismissed what she knew to be true about their son's challenges. And I remembered her feeling of relief when she received validation and support from our conversation.

"How is everything?"

"Well, Melissa, I don't know how to tell you this—"

I heard the crack in his voice.

"Karen is dead. Our son killed her."

I could not speak. I couldn't catch my breath. I couldn't believe what I was hearing on the other end of the phone, the heart-wrenching sobs of a man who had lost his wife, killed by the son they loved.

I tried to hold it together but began to cry uncontrollably.

"I'm so sorry. I can't even begin to know what to say. I'm just so sorry."

"Melissa, she was my best friend."

And he told me about the many years of their beautiful marriage and how they came to adopt Jesse.

"I need your help, please. The prosecuting attorney wants to try Jesse as an adult, although he's only fifteen," he said. "Jesse's attorney doesn't understand Jesse's disability and all of what Karen knew. He's a sweet boy—he didn't mean it. I know she would want him to get the support he needs. She loved him and he loved her."

"I will do whatever I can. Give the attorney my number and I'll find resources to help you. I'm so sorry."

Before I went to bed that night, I researched Karen's death, knowing it would have been reported by the news media. It was. The newspaper article I read said Karen and Jesse were watching an action-adventure movie together and something in it triggered his behavior.

And there it was, my fear confirmed. Not only can these kids morph into what they see, overstimulation of their brains can lead to violence.

What I also knew, more than anything else, was that Jesse had an accomplice to this crime.

He did not act alone.

His accomplice was society's ignorance of FASD.

Until FASD is understood, recognized, and diagnosed in the mental health community, more tragedies will take place, more innocent people will die, and people challenged with FASD will be put behind bars.

I was afraid to wake up in the morning; this nightmare wasn't going to go away.

Crying, I fell asleep.

Chapter 14

Jail Times Two

When I woke up my pillow was damp from sobbing throughout the night. Karen was dead. Her son was in jail and would be tried as an adult. Karen's husband needed my help, and I was to send him information about FASD and the criminal justice system so he could provide it to the attorney who would be representing Jesse. Still, it was a crapshoot if it would help his case.

I wanted to roll over and go back to the sleep that I didn't get during the night. My mind raced with thoughts of Jesse and Natalia in the same jail with the same disability. How could this happen!

After dragging myself into the kitchen to prepare a cup of coffee, I went to my basement office to email her husband the information. How heart-wrenching it must have been for him to visit his son in jail, trying to understand this disability and what triggered his son to kill. Just as Natalia was a victim of her disability, so was Jesse.

My thoughts wandered to Maurice. *Where was he now? How would he make it? Would he be caught in a life of crime because he was unable to get a correct diagnosis?* As I promised

Nicky that day of the conference over a year ago, I would find Maurice. Just as I began searching my computer for the attendance log, the phone rang.

"Hello?"

"Hi Mom. This is Natalia."

My heart was racing, pounding, about to jump from my chest into the phone.

"Natalia, how are you?"

"I'm okay, how are you? And how are Babushka and Nicky?"

Natalia was her usual self, even in jail. She was concerned, immediately asking about others. She had an incredible bond with her grandmother, who lived next door to us, whom she called Babushka, the Russian word for grandmother. Natalia's caring nature enabled her to be thoughtful and intuitive. She and her babushka cooked and sewed together. Their kindness to others was the glue, so to speak, that held their relationship close. However, Babushka's opinion of Natalia's friends was much different than Natalia's.

"Natalia, how long can you talk and what are they—"

"Mom, I don't have much time. I can make calls to you with a calling card that you need to set up. But, will you pay to get me out of here? I'm tired and scared."

"Natalia, are you pregnant?"

Hearing sniffling, I knew tears were beginning to flow.

"Yes, Mom. I found out while I was in Prince George's jail. I didn't drink, Mom. I promise, the baby is okay."

And there it was. One of my biggest fears. Would the

cycle of FASD continue and would this little baby become victimized by the same disability that had endangered Natalia's life?

Ironically, though she was in jail, I knew she was safe. Safe from the people she was hanging out with on the street, safe from the criminals who had stolen her identity, and safe from damaging her baby with the same toxic chemical, alcohol, that had wreaked havoc on her brain.

I needed to get in touch with her public defender to supply the information on FASD to give them an understanding of how and why she ended up behind bars. Suggestibility is a common trait of FASD. A person challenged with FASD will agree to most anything they are asked. She was vulnerable to the criminals who took advantage of her and would implicate her participation in the crime. In addition, she would have great difficulty understanding the extent of her participation and the consequences of her actions.

If I "sprang" her out of jail, she would run back to the street, finding the same trouble she had gotten herself into. For her safety, she needed to stay put while she and her attorney and I tried to make a plan for her safe return home. Knowing that all the charges against her might not be dropped, my hope was if they were not, the judge would intervene, requiring her to live in a group home, keeping her and the baby safe from her poor choices while she was on probation. She had a hand in this crime, but she was not the ringleader.

Her public defender would need as much information as possible, not just about Natalia's disability, but what led her to participate in this crime. Having kept meticulous notes about what had transpired over the past months, I would provide every piece of info I could to assist her.

Would things ever be normal again? At this point, it didn't matter. Natalia needed the courts to understand her disability, the baby needed to be safe, and Natalia wasn't getting out of jail anytime soon. The jail would be her home until she could safely return, if at all.

How many people inside the walls of that jail were impacted by an FASD? I had a feeling the numbers were probably staggering. Soon, I would be walking down the corridor of the jail, making my way to the little room where I would see Natalia sitting behind the glass wall. I couldn't help wondering what she had already experienced, what her baby had experienced, and what the future would hold.

Trying to keep my emotions in check, I realized I needed to conserve my energy to accomplish the work still ahead of me. Not just to help defend her from the crime at hand, but to defend her from the disability that had entrapped her.

Chapter 15

Jury Duty

Finishing up my now-cold cup of coffee and trying to get my head wrapped around the work of proving Natalia's innocence, it seemed the "to do" list was just getting longer and longer.

I hadn't checked my mailbox for a few days and was probably neglecting my own "to do" list. What could be waiting for me? Letters from creditors rejecting my credit because I was now connected to fraudulent activity?

When I opened the mailbox and grabbed the stack waiting for me, there was something from the state that looked pretty official. Good Lord, now what?

Jury summons.

Are you kidding me? Now of all times! I can't deal with jury duty. I could only imagine being interrogated by the attorneys, and I'm the only one in the room who raises my hand when they ask if anyone has an incarcerated family member because my daughter is a felon. Ha, they'll never pick me! That's one way to get out of it!

As I quickly opened the envelope, I saw the jury summons was not for me, but for Natalia. *ARE YOU KIDDING*

ME? In the past I've had to get her excused, had to send documentation of her disability. Living by the motto, "Never put off tomorrow what you can do today," I made a quick, or so I thought, phone call.

"Hello, I'm calling on behalf of my daughter about her summons for jury duty."

"Ma'am, is your daughter over the age of eighteen?"

"Yes."

"Well, ma'am, if she is over the age of eighteen, she will have to call in person."

I knew what I would have to do to prove her disability. The documentation that I'd have to dig through, copy, and provide on her behalf was far more than I had the energy for.

I blurted out to the woman on the line: "My daughter is *incarcerated.*" There, I said it. Clear, simply stated. My daughter is a jailbird, convict, inmate, prisoner, locked up, and not available for jury duty. *And she's pregnant!*

"Excuse me, ma'am? Did you say your daughter is in-carcerated—as in jail?"

"Yes, she is!" There, I said it again. "She has a mental disability, and I cannot put one more thing on my 'to do' list by sending you paperwork on her disability or her in-carceration for her jury duty to be waived."

There was a long pause, which was probably the clerk on the other end, covering the receiver to tell her office mates, "I've got a live one that beats all excuses to get out of jury duty."

Instead, it was the break that I needed.

She returned and said, "Ma'am, no problem, please don't worry about it. I'm removing her from our jury list."

Alleluia! Finally, someone understood!

Chapter 16

A Professional Pleader

And that's exactly what I needed: someone to understand.

Though I needed to talk to the public defender assigned to Natalia, my "go to" person was even better than that. I needed the person who had been there, done that, and understood the department of corrections because her own kids had been within the jail's walls. This person would navigate me through the process with expertise and compassion. There was nothing like another parent's perspective, and Anita was my "go to" person. She was also the mother of adopted children, some who were most likely impacted by FASD. She was a close friend, witty, candid, focused, and a stabilizing force. I couldn't allow myself emotional reactions during times like this, or I would find myself curled up into a ball, in tears!

Thankfully, Anita was a straight shooter, which might not be the best choice of words in the criminal world, though right on point. She understood far better than most how to navigate through challenging situations. Plus, she would take my call.

She picked up immediately and I explained the situation.

Anita was my informant. She methodically rattled off a whole lot of details as I frantically wrote them down:

Twenty-four hours in a holding cell, then released to the jail population. One call—twenty seconds. If she calls again, I can pay for a calling card, placing money on it to be used only for my phone number. Public defender gets assigned, then her prelimi-nary hearing is scheduled. Probably will plead guilty to first of-fense felony. Max won't be arrested unless Natalia gives up the information that he took her ATM card. There is no probable cause for his arrest because he did not access the ATM machine or teller. And be careful about the people they might meet in jail, the cellmates otherwise known as "bunkies." They will think they are their new best friend, then steer them in the wrong direction with their so-called experience and advice!

It was like getting the cheat sheet I needed, but I didn't want anything to do with it. And I certainly wouldn't want anyone to know I had it. Who wants to reveal their child is in jail for unexplained criminal behavior? I've heard it all: My boundaries were too loose, my boundaries were too tight, and they did it because of my poor parenting. Unless someone has walked in a caregiver's shoes, it is almost im-possible to understand the poor judgment of an FASD-impacted person. It's hard to get your brain wrapped around the reasoning they use.

Fortunately, neither of us cared much what the outside world thought about us or how we parented our kids. We focused on our kids, their challenges, and helping them.

I had what I needed from Anita and now I could make the

call to the public defender. I was praying this person would be open-minded about FASD while defending Natalia.

The public defender took my call and welcomed the timeline of events that led to Natalia's arrest. The attorney also showed interest in FASD, which she had never heard of. She gave me an indication of what to expect with the courts, preliminary hearings, arraignment, trial calendar, and what to expect with a "theft by taking" first offense felony case. Pretty much everything Anita had told me to expect. The attorney's professionalism, demeanor, and her willingness to be inundated with my crash course on FASD 101 were encouraging. She was a rule player and honest. Her client, Natalia, was her number one priority, and she would get Natalia's approval to keep me informed. Relieved, I ended the call.

I had a whole list of information to send. The timeline I'd sent to the detective on the case, security camera footage of the crimes, the bank transactions, Natalia's out-of-date diagnosis, assessments, literature on FASD and the criminal justice system, and the American Bar Association's resolution on FASD from William Edwards.

My conversations with the detective, Anita, and the public defender made me realize it would be very difficult to enter a not guilty plea for Natalia. As Anita had said, Max was out of the picture because there was no probable cause. He didn't use the ATMs or have contact with the teller, even though the video shows him sitting in the bank lobby. The criminals in the ATM security video and the company that owned the cab used as the getaway car would need to be positively identified and questioned. Although Natalia had willingly given the criminals her ATM card, she did not know how they were using it. She had been scammed, and it was going to be extremely difficult to prove it, especially because she was unwilling to point the finger at Max, who'd been equally duped by these criminals, to reveal his true part in this crime—talking Natalia into giving up her card. She seemed to prefer to take the fall, not realizing the seriousness of her actions and the consequences she would be facing, which was a common characteristic of FASD.

Throughout the next couple of days, the attorney and I exchanged emails and phone calls. She wanted an immediate evaluation from the clinic that worked with the mental health courts, which would help determine Natalia's mental health in relationship to her culpability of the crime. I needed to get an updated diagnosis for Natalia. Although not a diagnosis, FASD is the umbrella term for a range of effects that can result from prenatal alcohol exposure. Neurobehavioral Disorder Prenatal Alcohol Exposure (ND-PAE) is under this umbrella and is used by mental health professionals for diagnosis and insurance purposes as noted in the appendix of the Diagnostic Statistical Manual of Mental Disorders (DSM-5). I needed to contact and get the advice of the FASD expert and doctor who had contributed to ND-PAE's inclusion in the DSM-5. She and I had presented at the FASD conference held at the Georgia State Bar a few years earlier.

The conference was sponsored by the very same behavioral health and developmental disabilities agency that supported the clinic. This was the clinic that would be overseeing Natalia's mental assessment for the mental health courts. With the help of this FASD expert, the clinic that should be aware of FASD, and Natalia's psychiatrist, who had been caring for her since she was in elementary school, Natalia was sure to get resources and support from the courts.

When I researched the clinic that would assist the mental health courts with evaluating Natalia, I found nothing on FASD. This was troubling because many individuals with FASD end up in jail due to the effects of their "invisible disability." Had no one been listening at the FASD conference to then apply it to the mental health courts, especially at this clinic? And we wonder why the recidivism rate is so high when those arrested and jailed are on the spectrum but are never properly assessed and supported?

Nevertheless, the key players were all in place. At this point it was a waiting game, subject to the clinic staff understanding Natalia's diagnosis of ND-PAE (FASD), how it related to the facts of the case, and if she should, or would, be held accountable. Would Natalia be held accountable for her choices, despite the brain disorder that was due to alcohol in utero and was causing serious behavior challenges for her now, and possibly for the rest of her life?

As she was FASD-impaired and pregnant, the best I could hope for was that Natalia would be accepted into the mental health courts. The judge could also order her to be placed in a group home for expectant mothers and receive behavior management while on probation. I knew if Natalia didn't receive the help she needed in a group home, she was a flight risk. If she came home, she'd take off to find Max, putting herself and her unborn child at risk again.

There was one other possibility.

That would be if her dad got involved. Natalia didn't mention any involvement with him. I didn't ask, and her attorney didn't mention him either.

Over the course of the next couple of weeks, I met with Natalia, and we spoke about her future plans. She was still elusive about her role in the bank fraud, and her responsibility to be forthright about Max's involvement so her attorney could help her.

The preliminary court date had taken place, and now it was a matter of waiting for her evaluation from the mental health clinic as to whether she would be accepted or denied. Reading through their eligibility criteria, I thought Natalia seemed to meet the requirements, though it would probably be determined on a case-by-case basis. William Edwards was willing to talk with anyone in the mental health courts as well as her public defender. Billy understood FASD and knew what legal information might be needed to support Natalia's acceptance into their courts.

I was extremely hopeful and explained to Natalia this is what we would be aiming for. If they didn't accept her into their program, we would request the judge to court order her into a group home for expectant mothers.

On the off hours from visiting Natalia in jail, my trusted sidekick friend Diane and I visited various group homes for pregnant mothers, carefully interviewing the staff and making sure they would accommodate Natalia's needs. On one occasion, after interviewing and touring one of the group homes, we listened to a frightening spiel from one of the owners. Instinctively, we glanced at each other, knowing the place would be worse than jail. We gave each other that subtle look of "how fast can you run?" and took off toward the exit door, feeling like we were in a *Get Smart* episode where the doors were slamming shut around us. We were relieved to get out of there alive!

Thankfully, the other group homes we visited were adequate and would provide Natalia with a nurturing environment to teach her how to care for the baby while learning skills to manage her own life.

Her public defender now understood FASD and how it impacted Natalia's behavior choices. She would be Natalia's new best friend, not the "bunkie"! I let Natalia know she needed to listen to and cooperate with her attorney, who was her primary legal advocate. Natalia was not to seek the advice of her bunkie or anyone else who might be bending her ear in the wrong direction. It would be just the public defender and me meeting with Natalia.

So we thought!

Chapter 17

Let's Make a Deal

Every time I made the drive to visit with Natalia at the jail, it was surreal. I was thankful she was no longer living on the street, and relieved to know she was safe and would get the nutritional care needed for the baby. *And* no alcohol! I wasn't nervous about seeing her, only a bit nervous about driving to the jail. I was directionally challenged and didn't want to get lost on Atlanta's confusing roads. My ability to get lost, pull out a road map, and try to find my way back to the right path was always a joke in our family. Now, I was helping Natalia navigate her own road map of life.

When I arrived at the jail, the lobby was filled with people who were there to see those behind bars. I wondered about their stories and if their situations were as innocent, yet complicated, as Natalia's. As I signed in at the front desk, the clerk questioned my reason for being there. Holding back tears of frustration, I told her I was meeting my daughter. When the officer announced it was our allotted time for visitation, they took our car keys and herded us like cattle to the hallways. I was given directions on where

I was to go. I asked for some kind of building map to make sure I didn't get lost. They supplied one, which was a comfort, and I knew I wasn't the only one who needed help navigating through the jail's hallways. Who in this group had done this before and knew where they were going? Should I follow them . . . not a chance. Trusting only myself and my map, I'd find my way to Natalia.

Walking down the corridor, I tried to figure out which hallway would lead me to Natalia's visitation booth. It was like walking through a maze. I was unsure what turn to take as there was little signage. I knew the clock was ticking and any lost time would be time limited with Natalia.

As I got closer to the area where I would see Natalia, I could hear other visitors and inmates in their visitation booths. It was a kind of quiet screaming in frustration as the visitors addressed their family members-inmates. The frustration was real, and the anguish in the visitors' voices was emotionally charged. It's how I felt about Natalia, but I knew I didn't want our time spent rehashing her poor choices.

Taking a quick turn, I opened a door, only to reveal a short hallway with three more doors to choose from. *What was this?* It reminded me of the game show *Let's Make a Deal*, and I was to choose one of the doors for the prize that awaited me. But this was no game as I looked through each window, trying to find Natalia. Each booth had a glass divider with a small desk and vented speaker type of contraption. I would probably find her on one side, and I would be on the other.

As I looked beyond the glass divider, I could see the door she would enter to get into this small booth. People were walking around, but Natalia was not one of them and she was not in any of the booths.

Finally, I found the right booth and sat at a small desk facing the glass enclosure where Natalia would be sitting. The desk had graffiti etched on its surface. I didn't know how that was possible, as we weren't allowed to take any writing instruments into the visitation area. I waited, then she walked in, sat down, and I was numb. She looked good. All those things I wanted to say to her—asking her how she was feeling, why she didn't return home when she left, what was her plan once she got out, all these questions I had practiced in the car—were gone. Instead, emotions came pouring out, but I restrained them. I also understood why there was a glass panel between us. I wanted to reach out and shake some sense into her.

"Hi, Mom."

"Hi, Natalia. How are you doing?"

"I'm okay. How are Babushka and Nicky doing?"

She always asked about her grandmother and brother.

"Mom, will you get me out of here?"

And then she told me what it would take to bail her out, which I knew I wouldn't do. "Natalia, continue to listen and cooperate with your public defender. She understands your case better than your bunkie does and will do everything that's needed to help you."

"I will, Mom, but I really need you to get me out of here."

"I'll do the best I can, Natalia. I love you and want you safe. Your attorney is addressing the mental health courts for resources and support for you."

Hearing her begging me to get her out of the jail that was keeping her safe from the street was gut-wrenching. The feeling of knowing she was safer within these walls than outside them was so conflicting. I prayed for strength to know what to say to Natalia, to let her know I loved her. I could not lie and tell her I was posting bail to get her out, only that I would try my best to help her.

And that's all I could do.

Chapter 18

A Christmas Miracle

When I arrived home, I noticed Nicky was acting a little distant. The Christmas season was approaching, perhaps his work was becoming chaotic with holiday shoppers. Lately, he'd been a bit rebellious about doing his chores, though I believed it was unintentional. Over the years, I'd taught my children how to use calendars and schedules to keep them on task and organized. Concerned about Nicky's recent behavior, I looked at his calendar to see if he had been checking off his daily routines, which included his chores and work schedule. He had not. When this happens at home, something at work is usually going on. Prevention is key when caring for a person with FASD. I'd learned I had to stay at least two steps ahead of my children, noticing their demeanor and even reading their body language, to determine what they were having difficulty explaining. Their problem-solving skills are compromised, as is their ability to foresee that their behavior might affect others or cause problems—it's the challenge of understanding consequences.

I was planning on heading to the basement to get on my

computer and search for Maurice. I wanted to use the attendee list I'd received from the FASD conference where Nicky and I had met him, but the log was in an email attachment I hadn't been able to find. *Where the heck had I saved it?* I was trying to give myself a break for not remembering where it was in the confusing world of technology downloads. After all, I'd spent months now trying to find it when I wasn't searching for Natalia. I guessed it would have to wait, as I needed to address Nicky's recent attitude.

"Nicky, is everything okay?"

"Uh, uh, I don't know."

"What do you mean, you don't know?"

This was a big mistake on my part as "uhs" and "I don't knows" meant he's having difficulty processing information, stalling, and doesn't know how to share something that's uncomfortable for him to talk about it.

I needed to cut to the chase and help him find the words. Something was definitely going on at home and absolutely at work!

"Uh. Uh."

And then that look of frustration, distant and looking down.

"Okay, Nicky, I know something is going on at work because you are not on task here at home," I said. "Let's talk. Tell me and I'll help you."

"Mom, work is stupid. I do everything. I should be a manager. That's what the customers tell me. They give me everything to do and everyone else is on their phones not doing the work. The managers, too!" Nicky paused before continuing. "Ms. Jackson gives me too much and then I tell her I have a disability, and she said I don't and she says I have a bad attitude. I told her to look in my file, and I don't think she does. She tells me that she doesn't need to, and it's me not treating her with respect."

"Okay, she doesn't understand, Nicky, and it's time for us to have a talk with her to explain your disability."

With that, we left the house and drove to the store, which was about a fifteen-minute walk, but Nicky usually took thirty minutes. The walk is kind of his windup and wind down exercise and meditative time during the day. It's really good for him, as there are no distractions.

When we arrived, Ms. Jackson, the front-end manager, and her manager were standing at the entrance of the store.

"Hi, Ms. Jackson, do you have a moment?"

I had spoken to her before but not in this context.

"Yes, I can talk. Nicky, did you tell your mom what happened? Why did you do that? We took care of it."

I interrupted her. "Ms. Jackson, I'm just here to help clarify a few things to help you understand Nicky's behavior."

"Oh, I understand his behavior," she replied. "Nicky, why did you go home and tell your mother?"

Nicky, speechless and needing help, looked at me.

"Ms. Jackson, did you read his file?"

She gave Nicky a stern look and turned back to me.

"Ms. Jacobus, I know all about his file."

Pausing, I caught my breath, as this scenario was all too

familiar. Ms. Jackson needed to understand FASD, and this might not be pretty.

"But did you read his file? Because if you did, you would understand that Nicky also has an anxiety disorder. He was afraid you were going to fire him, so he came home to tell me."

Things were getting a little heated with her defensiveness and confusion about Nicky's challenges. It was evident we needed to find an office for privacy.

We sat down with another manager, who was aware of Nicky's challenges, but only observed the meeting. I handed some educational material about FASD to Ms. Jackson. She put it aside without acknowledging it. I explained that FASD is an "invisible disability" that goes undetected and can be misinterpreted as willful behavior when an individual with FASD becomes overwhelmed from trying to follow too many instructions or taking on too many responsibilities. I asked her what had led up to the problem.

She told me Nicky had been working on a register but was pulled off to temporarily help another manager in another department. As Nicky was heading to help the other manager, yet another manager stopped him. In the meantime, Ms. Jackson wondered where he was and saw him walking in the store (he was most likely walking from one department to another) and questioned why he wasn't back at the register. He tried to explain this to her, which he had difficulty processing, and she questioned him again. At this point, he shut down and stopped talking.

I explained to her that at that point, Nicky had entered a state of confusion, frustration, anxiety, and panic. His adaptive behaviors are challenged, and when he's settled into a job he is doing, then given a multitude of jobs to complete at the same time, his coping mechanism is to shut down. His brain was not going to work correctly. What often happened next is his frustration would work its way into what looks like a bad attitude. Those impacted by FASD can also have difficulty regulating their emotions, which in turn can escalate into explosive behavior. Thankfully, Nicky shuts down as a coping mechanism. He doesn't demonstrate explosive behavior . . . yet! Many kids with FASD have to work hard to avoid acting out their frustration. And, quite frankly, the typical adult has difficulty with this also.

"Ms. Jackson, in the situation you described, Nicky is working far beyond his abilities in trying to handle all that was given to him. To have several managers pulling him in many directions when his brain has just settled on the register work is extremely difficult," I said. "And I guarantee you that as he's making his way from one department to the next, customers are asking him for help finding items in the store."

Nicky looked at me with relief, nodding his head.

"Just hearing from you about what Nicky was required to do, especially in this situation, makes my head spin. Now, take the customers who need Nicky's help into consideration, and that makes me want to run!"

There was little response.

"I understand your lack of awareness about FASD. It's a difficult disability to comprehend since he looks completely capable. Please read this information. It should help you, and if there's anything you think of that would better help Nicky with his job, please let us know."

Perhaps she was embarrassed, didn't believe he had a disability, or just didn't have time for it. Regardless, Nicky's job was secure. The information about his disability was in his file. He wasn't going to be fired.

As we were leaving the store, one of Nicky's customers stopped to talk with him. The customer was disappointed Nicky wasn't working that day and asked when he was going to be the store manager because Nicky seemed to run the store and was always helpful.

We said good-bye to the customer, and as we turned to leave, we saw Ms. Jackson standing behind us.

She had overheard the customer, smiled, and walked back into the store. I wonder if she *really* understood. Fortunately for us, a few weeks later she moved to another store.

When I got back home and was beginning to search my computer for the attendance log that would lead me to Maurice, the phone rang. It was Barbara, who lived a few houses away. Just the voice I needed to hear. Barbara was amazing in every way. She was a spiritual breath of fresh air, and her entire family had a sense of humor that could break the monotony of any gloomy day.

Ironically, she and her adult daughters cared for foster children in her home. Many of the children were challenged with multiple disabilities, which included suspected FASD. Not only did she offer these children a family, safety, and hope, her care was impeccable, and the love she showed was unmistakable. Barbara's family had their own personal challenges with the health of a family member, but they had unbreakable faith. Her daughter Kimberly, who was an angel in her own right, struggled with sickle cell anemia. I was fortunate enough to also form a friendship with Kimberly that I treasured. She had been hospitalized much of the year, and her strength was beyond what I could imagine. When I needed to pull myself out of my own difficulties, I reflected on Kim. She is smart, beautiful, and an inspiration.

As Barbara and I spoke, she heard the exhaustion in my voice.

"Okay, girl, you can't fool me. What's going on?"

"Just a little tired, Barbara. I've been with Nicky at his work, talking to his managers; all is okay now."

"*And?*"

"Well, I'm trying to find Maurice. Remember I had told you about him at the conference that I attended with Nicky? Maurice is challenged with an FASD and will most likely be living on the street because he's aged out of foster care. I need to find him."

"Melissa, you will find him. Can we pray for a moment?"

And then, over the phone, Barbara began to pray. An

amazing, heartfelt, spiritual prayer, a deepening of love and hope that spoke to my soul. It was a prayer asking for God's grace and His help finding Maurice. It was detailed with the purest intent.

As I wiped my eyes and thanked Barbara, she told me that Kimberly was back in the hospital. That is Barbara, praying I would find a young man I didn't even know, as her daughter was in the hospital again, needing prayers of her own. There was no shortage of prayers from Barbara; she is one of God's angels. As we hung up, I told her I'd make a visit to the hospital.

I took a deep breath and put Barbara's prayer in action. I headed for the computer to begin searching for Maurice as I had started out to do that morning. I dreaded searching for the attendance log. For months, I had searched every possible file. As the computer was warming up, I kept reflecting on Barbara's prayer. I signed in and clicked on my "important" files, about ten files from the FASD file, which is where I should have put it.

There it was! Trembling, I clicked it open. It was intact, and I printed out the log. As I reviewed every name in detail with titles/organizations noted, I found Maurice. He had listed himself with several titles and several organizations but no phone number or email address. Still, what he had listed was a place to start.

As I thought of Maurice, I was so thankful Nicky was still safe at home until I was able to provide safe interdependence through supportive housing of some sort.

For now, the lead to find Maurice had been found! Prayers were answered. Thank you, God, and His angel Barbara!

It was a Christmas miracle!

Chapter 19

Baked Potato in a Bag

The Christmas miracle seemed to be short-lived. Not being in the Christmas spirit, I had not decorated the house as usual. Instead, I only hung the Christmas stockings my children had since they arrived from Russia. Each stocking was a little bit different so they could easily identify theirs. These Russian Christmas stockings had a special place on the fireplace mantel, and each Christmas morning they would be filled with simple little treats. Exploring their contents would be the first order of business before church and breakfast.

Angry and heartbroken over what was happening, I was not able to hang up Natalia's stocking.

My thoughts of Natalia and her Merry Little Band of Misfits in jail continued. Her bunkie's influence was reflected in what Natalia was telling me—they'd made promises to meet up after they both got out of jail, and her bunkie was giving her misleading legal guidance, which wasn't at all helpful for someone who was already in jail due to her poor judgment. Natalia might have been morphing into her bunkie, but at least she wasn't on the street. FASD-challenged people reflect their environment. It's the very reason keeping their boundaries safe and secure is so important. Home was safe.

But still, my thoughts swirled around the attitudes and behaviors she would imitate. As they say, "birds of a feather flock together." At this point, many of those birds were vultures, living off the remains of street culture. I didn't want Natalia to be eaten alive. She certainly would have been, had she continued living on the street.

Trying to give her happy reminders of home while she was in jail, I created and mailed photo postcards of her from earlier special occasions—our traditions of celebrating birthdays, Christmas, and even one of her making her First Holy Communion, reminding her that God wouldn't give up on her!

I hoped seeing photos of these celebrations would remind her of the love that surrounded her. I hoped she would remember how it was at home on the "outside," so she wouldn't end up "inside" again.

Of all our family's celebrations, Natalia loved Christmas the most. She was a huge help during the holidays because she was our primary Christmas interior decorator. Detailed and talented! Every year the same Christmas decorations were placed in the same location in each room. After the holidays, all the decorations were organized in bins marked for the appropriate room and stored. It made it easy to decorate. All consistent, organized, and simple. Keeping life organized for the kids eased the challenges of

FASD, eliminating the overwhelming stress that clutter can cause. So decorating and holidays were a fun time to enjoy, and we did! Natalia was great at it, always adding her special touch and her delicious Christmas desserts. She is gifted at both!

Christmastime was wrapped in traditions, and one of our favorites was the "Santa Phantom" of the twelve days of Christmas. Our dear friends Molly and Steve, who had tutored our children and were among the first of our friends to truly understand FASD, began this tradition with us. In December, we would select a family and secretly drop off simple presents, along with a poem, every day for the twelve days leading up to Christmas. After our twelve days of adventure, we revealed ourselves. We had fun, and so did the recipients, many of whom paid it forward the next year. We all agreed it was much more meaningful to be on the giving end. And for years, it was a tradition that was extremely meaningful to our family. A few years earlier, Natalia, dressed in a Santa hat and beard, had been the incognito delivery elf for one of these families.

While Natalia was sitting in jail, would she reflect on the tradition of the Santa Phantom? The giving of the season being more important than the getting? Would she have an opportunity to celebrate Christmas and God's gifts? I prayed she would at least remember the past and the love that surrounded our family. It was still there, just a much different surrounding for her.

Even though I wasn't feeling much like celebrating the

Christmas season, Nicky deserved to enjoy it. He wanted no part of Natalia's issues or reminders of her behaviors. He often would say this situation was her choice, not his. Why did he have to pay the price for her decisions with me spending *all* my time trying to help her? And he was partly right, as his Christmas season was affected.

Thinking it would put me in the Christmas spirit, I put on Christmas music. The phone rang. It was the jail and would I accept the charges. Of course, I would.

"Hi, Mom. Merry Christmas."

"Hi, Natalia. How are you?"

"I'm okay. I was just wondering what you were doing for Christmas? Did you do the Santa Phantom this year?"

"No, Natalia, we were a little preoccupied. Couldn't quite get the time to write the poems and come up with the gifts to deliver. Plus, Santa's main delivery elf wasn't available. It's not the same." *Maybe next year*, I thought.

"I'm sorry, Mom."

"So, Natalia, what are you doing? Does the jail serve a Christmas meal?"

"I don't know if they'll do anything, but my bunkie and several other girls and I have planned a Christmas snack."

"That sounds interesting. What are you all planning?"

"Well, we've been saving our snacks throughout the week, like the coffee mocha packs, candy bars, and a girl is making Rice Krispies treats out of food she's been collecting. I'm making 'baked potato in a bag.'"

"What's 'baked potato in a bag'?"

"It's where I take potato chips in a bag and add hot water. Then when the potato chips are soft, you mush them up and it tastes like a baked potato," Natalia said. "It's going to be fun. We're all trying to have our own Christmas together in here."

Trying to make the best out of the situation, I believed she was missing home a bit, and God willing, realizing that she needed to change her ways so she didn't end up in jail again.

Her time on the call was about to end. "Mom, I have to get off the phone. Please tell Nicky and Babushka 'Merry Christmas' for me. Love you."

"Merry Christmas, Natalia. Enjoy your Christmas snack and the baked potato in a bag. Love you, too! Let's talk when you get a chance again."

"Okay, Mom. Merry Christmas."

I walked over to the mantel and hung up her Christmas stocking.

Chapter 20

It's a New Year

The Christmas holidays were uneventful. I guess that was a good thing given the year's events. I was thankful Natalia was safe, and her attorney seemed to have a solid understanding of Natalia's challenges with FASD and was trying to accommodate her needs after she was released from jail, whenever that would be. I prayed the mental health court would accept her into its treatment program and supervise her probation, which would keep her and the baby safe. If not, the backup plan was the group home under the court's order. Knowing these options allowed me a tiny reprieve from the stress of the unexpected.

It was New Year's Day and Natalia called, seeming to be missing home a little bit. She wanted to know what we were doing for the day, asking me if Nicky and I were going to have our traditional New Year's dinner of Russian food, which included all of her favorites: borscht, pelmeni, cucumber salad, and a Russian cake purchased at the Russian deli. This was another indication that, perhaps, she was longing for the comfort of family. She told me about the nice security guard on their floor who turned up the television at midnight so the girls on the hall could hear when the ball dropped at midnight in New York's Times Square. Natalia could see the TV from her cell and was thankful to have had that privilege.

I was talking with her about the option of the group home for pregnant women if the mental health courts did not accept her diagnosis. The one we'd selected was highly respected and a great backup plan. The group home would help her care for her baby while providing Natalia with job training or furthering her education. We would wait to hear from the courts.

Natalia was distracted and a bit detached on the phone. I could sense something was wrong. I needed to plan a visit to see her. Her visitation hours were limited, and I wasn't getting the allotted time to see her. So, who was?

Then her frequent phone calls stopped, and my gut instinct got stronger. Something was terribly wrong. *Why wasn't I hearing from her? Who could be bending her ear?*

Natalia's public defender sent me an email. The news was not good.

The mental health court had denied Natalia. There was no appeal, as the team had total discretion.

Furious with their lack of using the "case-by-case situation" as stated in their criteria for acceptance into the program, I again wondered if this is why recidivism was so high in the jail population! If they recognized FASD and learned how to intervene with a treatment plan, maybe their numbers in the prison population wouldn't be so staggering!

Still, I tried to give the mental health courts the benefit of the doubt, as it seemed their decision reflected their lack of FASD knowledge. They weren't educated on FASD, and when this was all over, I would make it my goal to make sure that they were! No one should ever be denied help because a system is uninformed.

Natalia's attorney's email was direct but compassionate. She understood what was needed, was a quick study with FASD, and was navigating Natalia's best interests through this broken system. Her focus now was getting Natalia the strategies and accommodations needed to give her the best possible outcome as soon as she was out of jail and released to the group home. The attorney was spot-on with what was needed. She was committed to Natalia and concerned about her welfare in the future. She was doing all she could to ensure Natalia was returned to a safe community environment.

The attorney would be breaking the bad news to Natalia on their next visit. She worked well with Natalia, and this information was to be addressed between the two of them. Using her legal advice, and at her discretion, I would then step in to talk with Natalia, guiding her to the next healthy step for her future at the group home, where they would continue to give her prenatal help, parenting classes, life skills, and supervise her probation. All this would be included in the terms of probation. The court date had not been set, but the process was moving quickly. We would need to make sure all requirements were in place for her release into the group home.

Early afternoon the next day, Natalia called me unexpectedly. I was relieved to finally hear from her.

"Hi, Mom. I know about the mental health court and that they didn't accept me into their program."

"Natalia, I am so sorry about that. It's going to be okay. The courts are aware of the group home for pregnant girls, and your attorney is working on accommodating the terms of your probation to include them."

"Mom, I'm not going to a group home. I'm going to live with Pop. He told me everything. He is going to get me out of here as soon as possible. I'll sleep on his couch, have a job, and take care of the baby."

I was shocked at what I was hearing.

"Natalia, when have you been talking to Pop?"

"Um, he has been coming in with his girlfriend since I got in jail."

At this point I was seeing *red*!

"And you think things are going to be better for you with Pop instead of the group home where they will look after you and the baby and teach you life skills for your future?"

"Mom, they will have rules I'll have to follow. Pop won't have those kinds of rules. Why do you sound so disappointed?"

Disappointed?! Luckily, Natalia couldn't see me because I was steaming with anger from every part of my body and about to explode.

"I'm more in shock that you are making this choice! Pop

didn't come into the courts and sprinkle fairy dust on everything to lessen the terms of your probation. Your attorney has worked hard, acting on your behalf and communicating with me to help you with the accommodations needed for you and the baby. What happened with your being upset when Pop went to the beach as you were trying to get your money from him?"

"Um, I don't know. I haven't thought about it. Plus, he said he will pay my fines with my money that he kept. He said he and his girlfriend are going to buy a house in Florida, and I can move in with them. They've been nice to me and aren't as serious as you are. I don't want to live with a bunch of girls anyway."

Nothing she was saying at this point made any sense. But, boy, it made sense to her. *Nonsense* was what it was! A house in Florida, sure, that will go over well with the terms of her probation since she won't be allowed to leave the state of Georgia without the court's approval.

"Well, let me tell you, Natalia. This is serious, and you need to think about protecting your baby. The group home will help you prioritize your life with the baby. If you are not in a safe environment to help you and supervise your probation correctly, you will be back in jail. Is that where you want to end up again?"

Natalia laughed, and I could sense her attitude of entitlement. Her comments were becoming flippant and aloof. The conversation was over, and I could only hope that her attorney could reason with her. *Good God, what was I saying?*

Natalia was impulsive and reasoning was not at the forefront of her brain. Nothing was at the forefront, except most likely finding her boyfriend, Max.

"Mom, I can't talk anymore. I have to get off the phone 'cause my time is up. I think my court date will be next week 'cause Pop told me he's getting me out of here real soon."

We ended the call.

This was a frustrating new development that needed to be addressed. The attorney and I had agreed that jail was a relatively safe place for Natalia until she was released to the group home. Based on this new information, I was concerned that living with her father would not be the best solution, and Natalia would be right back on the street.

Due to her FASD challenges, she didn't understand the long-term consequences that awaited her. If she left his care, she would not have enough supervision to keep her on track without violating her probation or her getting in trouble again.

It was clear that for her benefit, the terms of her probation needed to be revisited with the understanding that she most likely would not be correctly supervised and would be back on the street.

That afternoon, I got an email from Natalia's attorney saying that she had spoken to Natalia about her sentencing. She would be released once the jail received the sentencing order. Her court date would be set for the following week.

It was a very long week. There was nothing I could do

since the decision had been made that Natalia would be released into her father's care. He really didn't know what kind of mess he was about to step into because he never acknowledged her FASD disability.

When we were married, he didn't attend our children's psychological assessments, didn't acknowledge their intellectual deficits (which weren't caused by not trying harder), and he didn't read the FASD information that I provided him. Their adaptive functioning of navigating life's choices was compromised. Many times their actions would look like rebellion or emotional outbursts (tantrums). These can be a by-product of behavior issues, due to their inability to self-regulate when overwhelmed. "Shutting down" is another coping mechanism for being overwhelmed. If one has ever witnessed the emotional outbursts, shutting down would be preferred. However, then the behavior is not addressed and sneaky behavior might be just around the corner.

Any of these behaviors can basically be described as taking moodiness to a whole new level.

These behaviors could look believable to people who didn't enroll in the FASD 101 course. It could seem the children were willfully making poor choices, when in reality FASD had diminished their ability to make good choices, unless strong boundaries and supportive measures were in place. Again, it's not because they won't—it's because they can't. If caregivers simplify their environment with structure, routine, and protective factors, those with an FASD are more likely to have success in making good choices.

The "honeymoon" stage of taking Natalia in would be short-lived. Her attorney and others who understood Natalia's challenges realized it would result in a mess, and bets were being taken for when the honeymoon stage would end.

Chapter *21*

A Broken System

The mood was solemn in court that day. The courtroom was filled with people sitting and waiting to hear the outcome of their loved ones' cases. Would they be sentenced or released on probation? Natalia was getting out. Going from the frying pan into what could possibly be the fire, without a fire extinguisher.

I took a seat behind Natalia's dad while we waited for Natalia's case to be heard. If the opportunity presented itself, I had material about FASD ready to give to the judge or the probation officer. Natalia's dad was rustling papers, organizing his paperwork, then turned around and asked me if I had brought Natalia's passport and other identification documents as he had demanded earlier. Knowing that important original documents would inevitably get lost in the wrong hands, I had not brought them with me. When I explained this to him, he quickly fired back that I was just going to make it hard on them.

He mentioned that Natalia hated Max, and there was no way she would be in touch with him, nor would she have access to the internet to find him. He added that he despised Facebook, and it would not be allowed. Despite this, I was concerned Natalia would still have unsupervised access to the internet and would continue to be at risk. During my visits with Natalia while she was in jail, she had told me a different story about her relationship with Max. She intended to find him once she was released. She was conning her dad and because he didn't understand her disability and the supervision she needed, it was just a matter of time before he would find out.

I relayed her relationship with Max to him, praying he would have a change of heart about the group home for girls that had been lined up for her; instead, he scoffed at it.

As he began to turn around to face the judge's chambers, Natalia walked into the courtroom with a swagger, snickering as she kept her eyes on the floor.

We both looked at her.

He commented in disgust, "Look at her. Now she has an attitude she learned in there. This is why she needs to get out. Her attitude is not going to fly with me!"

I didn't dare comment this could easily be behavior she learned from the street, and it was also a coping mechanism.

As the judge addressed Natalia and her attorney, Natalia's sentencing was revealed: First Offender/Conditional Discharge, Guilty-Felony-Theft by Taking, four years of probation, restitution to be paid to the bank and court, and community service. They were asked if Natalia understood the sentencing and the terms of the probation. She agreed and was sent out of the courtroom to sign the discharge papers, with an understanding that the conditions of probation included "no contact with persons or places of disreputable or harmful character," meaning her boyfriend, Max.

Leaving the courtroom and walking into the lobby, I overhead Natalia's dad confronting the attorney, asking why she didn't plead down Natalia's sentencing further. The attorney knew Natalia needed the supervision of the court's probation terms if she wasn't going to have close supervision in her new environment. The attorney walked toward me, and I thanked her for all the help she had given Natalia.

I found the court's chief probation officer and handed him Natalia's diagnosis and FASD literature that pertained to the criminal justice system.

His comment after reading the literature was one of mixed emotions, asking me if Natalia's diagnosis was addressed in the mental health courts. More staggering was his comment that this information could apply to many of those on probation. He had never heard of FASD and asked if he could keep the handouts for future reference.

There was nothing more I could do about the outcome of Natalia's case, but I would make a case with the mental health courts to offer an FASD training seminar in the near future. This broken system needed to change—to help Natalia, and those who were sure to be back in jail without proper assistance.

Before leaving the courthouse, I thanked Natalia's attorney again. We agreed our hands were tied, and neither of us felt confident Natalia was out of harm's way.

Not knowing when I would see Natalia again, I prayed God would watch over her and keep her safe. I also knew that Natalia's dad and his girlfriend would experience a few of Natalia's unmanageable challenges, the CliffsNotes version, before real chaos erupted.

Although I wondered when I would get her call for help, I certainly didn't expect the call that came soon thereafter.

Chapter 22

Revelation

About six weeks after Natalia had been released to her dad's care, the phone rang. Natalia's dad wanted to know the name and phone number of the group home for pregnant girls I had tried to set up for Natalia upon her release from jail.

"What are you talking about? I'm a bit confused," I said. "What's going on? Where's Natalia?"

"She's with me, getting checked into a hotel."

I reminded him the group home would have been set up through the courts, and there was a waiting list. Natalia would have to have been accepted into the home before being placed on probation.

He said he screwed up.

Well, that was a revelation.

"I never should have taken her out of jail. She's been plotting, emailing, and on Facebook with Max—behind my back! Who does she think she is? She's violated my trust."

I kept my response to myself. But I was thinking:

Really, you don't say. You let her on the internet and didn't expect that she'd go looking for him? Just because you thought

*she should follow your rules, you really thought she would?
You've got to be kidding me!*

*She needed CLOSE SUPERVISION! And I wanted to shout
from the top of my "overprotective," sheltering, motherly helicopter voice: I TOLD YOU SO!*

"I've given her a place to live, baby items, a job at the
company, and what does she do? Puts me and everyone at
risk! How can she not understand the consequences of her
rotten choices of ruining her life by getting in touch with
her lousy boyfriend? She's getting a second chance . . . how
can she throw it away? Does she not get it?"

*Am I hearing what I think I'm hearing? Should I play the tape
recorder back on what he should understand or play the tape forward on what we all knew was her future if she wasn't closely
supervised with protective factors?*

*Well, no, she doesn't get it. That's why she's making these
poor choices! Though she's chronologically twenty-one years old,
her emotional development is delayed. Would you not watch a
fifteen-year-old closely, preventing them from finding trouble?
Do you want to read all her psych evals now? They might come
in handy!*

"She has no guilt or remorse. I'm done with her. I'm
dropping her off at an extended-stay motel near the jail!"

Knowing Natalia was already in contact with her boyfriend and possibly his hoodlum friends, having her come
back to the house with Nicky at home was not an option.
But she was also eight months pregnant.

"No, don't drop her off. Bring her back to your house

and I'll stay with her during the day when you're at work, and you stay with her at night," I pleaded. "Just until the baby's born and then we'll revisit the situation. Please don't drop her off at the motel. We can figure this out."

"Nope, I'm already here. Not keeping her for another minute. I'll pay for a few nights' stay and then she's on her own. She's chosen this. I was here to help her, but she wants Max. I'm done!"

He sounded frustrated, distraught, and disgusted. I wish he had followed the attorney's advice. Some caregivers get it, some don't, and some are in denial.

He said, "I'm at the motel. The hospital is down the street. Got to go."

"Wait, what's the address of the motel—I need the room number, too, and Natalia needs food."

And with that he hung up and called me a short time later to give me the motel address and her room number. He said Natalia took only a small amount of clothes shoved into her purse: nothing more, leaving everything behind. This was an indication to me that she would be on the move, not staying long at the motel and certainly not carrying a bunch of stuff from one location to the next while she's pregnant.

Quickly, I got on my computer to look up the motel and directions. I knew I needed to find her, get her enough food for weeks, and clothing items to get her to set up at "home" at the motel until she had the baby. If not, God knows where the baby would be delivered!

As I was researching the motel, I saw an email from the attorney asking me if I had heard from Natalia's dad. Apparently, he had contacted her to find out what it would take to put Natalia back in jail. I guess he had a change of heart about taking her out of jail too soon. A little bit too late! There she had shelter, food, and supervision to help her when she went into labor.

I called Natalia and told her I would come by to check on her. She didn't want me to come and said Max was on his way from DC. She was fine and would stay put. It was March and still a bit cold outside. Because her dad had paid for her motel room for a few days, it brought some relief as I knew she had a place to stay until I could try to convince her to come home. I also let the motel management know she was eight months pregnant and alone.

I called her again several days later. I told her I was going to be in the area at the courthouse and would come by to see her. Although she was making up excuses to avoid me, she should have known I would be there, regardless. It was apparent Max had not arrived, and as odd as it may sound, I would rather have had him with her when she went into labor. I didn't want her to be alone. Because of her limited self-awareness, my bet was she would ignore the labor pains, and the baby would be born in the motel room without medical care, putting her and the baby in danger.

I arrived at the motel and called the front desk and asked them to ring Natalia's room.

"Hi, Natalia. How about we go to lunch, then shop for some food for you? I'm in my car in the parking lot."

"Mom, I'm doing laundry."

"Natalia, do your laundry later. Let's go to the Walmart down the street and get you some clothes and food. I'm not leaving until I see you, plus I'm hungry!"

"Okay, Mom. I'm on my way down."

Seeing her, my tears were held back by the wall of frustration I was feeling that she had left the jail with her dad, then pulled the stunt to get in touch with Max.

Having her cornered in the car, she had to listen as we drove to the store.

"Natalia, this is not a good situation for you or the baby. You are her best bet in life to keep her safe. Is this how to do it? Living in a motel, hoping Max is going to show up? Come home with me or let me at least take you to the group home where they will help you."

Though I wasn't sure the group home would have an opening, she could stay with me until they did—buying some time to make sure Natalia and the baby were safe with the impending delivery.

"No, Mom. I'm going to wait for Max. He's on his way. I can't believe Pop dumped me off at this motel. He went to the homeless shelter, and they couldn't take me until Monday. He told them that was fine, and we'd be back on Monday. Then he drives to this motel, pays for a few nights, hands me a couple of twenties, and said don't call me when you get back in jail. How could he do that?"

145

"It sounds horribly hurtful, but he also thought he was helping you when he took you out on probation. He gave you a place to live, food, help for you and the baby, and a job, then behind his back, you're contacting Max. You lied to him and you lied to me at the jail. It all catches up to you! It's done now. Do you want to come home with me?"

"No, Mom. I'm waiting for Max."

"Natalia, I just want to scoop you up and bring you home. You need to call me if you need anything! I can't make your decisions for you, but I'm here for you. Even after undermining me at the jail. I love you and want you safe. Call me for anything."

We grabbed some lunch and went to the Walmart to pick up groceries. I continued to load up on whatever I thought she would eat and bought enough to carry her over for a few weeks. We shopped for clothes and toiletries, which this motel wasn't going to provide. I hoped supplying her with the comforts of home would help make this her new home for the next couple of weeks. I insisted she call me when she thought she was going into labor.

Driving back to the motel, we were quiet, which was unusual as I usually have a lot to say. I felt like I had used up all my words, and there was nothing more I could say that would change her mind. We prayed, and I helped her bring her groceries into the musty room that smelled of cigarettes. We hugged and I left.

I was relieved that she was alive, frustrated that she

wouldn't come home, and prayerful that this situation was in God's hands again.

I went to the motel lobby and paid an extra week on her room. I told the motel clerk if he heard moaning coming from Room 314 to call 911.

And ask them to send a midwife.

Chapter 23

Foster Care

A few weeks after Natalia's dad left her at the motel, he called me saying he was going to contact the hospital where she was receiving prenatal care to alert them about her new living situation. I was pleased he was following through with a bit of her care. However, he also said he had canceled the company health insurance for Natalia and had requested that the hospital assign a social worker to her. I prayed the social worker would reapply for Medicaid for Natalia and her baby. Natalia's dad then asked me for any medical or psych evaluations concerning Natalia. I had mixed feelings about this, but I sent the information to him, thinking he would use it in Natalia's best interests so the medical professionals helping her would better understand her diagnosis and interventions to help her.

Despite her challenges with FASD, Natalia was gentle, loving, and had the ability to recalibrate her choices into healthy ones for herself and her unborn baby if she were living in a stable environment with protective factors. However, if she had consumed alcohol before she knew she was pregnant, there was a possibility that her baby would be impacted by FASD, and she would need services for her newborn. Still, she would want to do what was right for her baby, and I wanted everything possible done right for Natalia. She had not caught up to her chronological age, and her emotional age was more like that of a teenager. I believed the hospital's postpartum programs and social worker would assess her situation and either guide Natalia in parenting classes or take other measures by contacting the state's family and children services after the baby was born.

Three weeks later, at the end of March, Natalia gave birth. The hospital was equipped with Natalia's history and what the future looked like for the two of them.

Although I was praying that the baby, a girl, would be kept with Natalia upon leaving the hospital, shortly thereafter, she was placed in foster care.

Understanding that foster care will do everything possible to keep families together was my only solace, as it was an extremely lengthy process. "All" Natalia had to do was follow their directions, attend the court hearings, parenting classes, the recommendations they made, and within time she would be reunited with her daughter. That would be the most logical decision, if Natalia could manage it. But what if she couldn't manage it?

The foster care system needed to know about her ND-PAE (FASD) diagnosis to understand that her arrest and subsequent time in jail were due to her disability, and she needed interventions to help her.

However, despite months of countless calls and emails, foster care offered me little to no response, and when they did respond, it was with a runaround. I could only imagine they were overworked and underpaid, though that was no consolation to me for the way Natalia and her baby's case was being mishandled. I wanted to see the baby and visit with the foster parents as soon as possible.

I hadn't heard from Natalia's dad after he said he contacted the hospital, except that he was washing his hands of the whole mess and was done with it all.

And although I'd heard from Natalia a few times, I had no idea where she was living.

I continued to try to get some answers from foster care about the case and the baby's whereabouts. A caseworker finally let me know I would only get the information by being present in the courtroom at juvenile court for the "deprivation trial," or review of the case. I hadn't been informed of previous court dates because I wasn't seeking custody of the baby. In what seemed to be a slip, the caseworker revealed this was the third court hearing to take place. Natalia and Max had been present at one and missed the other. They had not been consistently visiting the baby. With a history like this, their parental rights would be terminated if they didn't show they were actively seeking to be joined with her. However, for people with FASD, adhering to a schedule is extremely difficult. They cannot navigate schedules without an "environmental prescription" of support and someone to help manage it.

The day of the hearing, the hallway outside the court-room was like a three-ring circus. It wasn't just their case being heard but many other families caught up in the system due to their own choices or undiagnosed disabilities.

My work was cut out for me as I scanned the room to figure out who the players were. I was shocked that the first player I spotted was Natalia's dad. A woman was holding onto his arm, and they were speaking to people I thought might be social workers. I'd not met this woman and thought this was going to be an interesting introduction. As I walked toward them, I bumped into another familiar face, an adoption attorney. We had worked on a FASD advocacy board together to bring greater awareness to FASD years earlier. We spoke briefly, catching up on the past few years, then he dropped the ball when he revealed who he was representing. He said he was working on a case for a couple to get custody of their daughter's baby.

It was Natalia's daughter and his client was Natalia's dad.

"Are you telling me you are working with him?" I said as I glanced toward DS, who was only a few feet away.

"Yes, you know him?"

"Yes. While you and I were working on bringing about FASD awareness, he and I were in the middle of a divorce. Our daughter is impacted by FASD, and her baby may be as well. He didn't believe our kids had a disability. He thought they needed to try harder and make better choices."

I wanted to share some background information with him while I had the chance and was far away from eavesdroppers. "The baby must be cared for by someone who understands her needs. And if my daughter can get the help she needs, she should be with her daughter, if she so chooses."

The adoption attorney and I were deep in conversation about FASD and the work we had accomplished with still so much to be done when DS and his companion walked up to us.

Interrupting our conversation, the woman said, "Well, I guess I'm the only one who doesn't know you."

I reached out my hand and introduced myself. "I'm Melissa, Natalia's mom. This attorney and I worked together years ago on the board of the Georgia National Organization of Fetal Alcohol Syndrome and for an event called 'Pregnancy Pause,' where a woman pauses from drinking alcohol during her nine months of pregnancy."

Without skipping a beat, the attorney and I continued talking the FASD language for a few more minutes. Realizing it might be a conflict of interest to be talking with him, as he had evidently been hired by Natalia's dad, I excused myself.

I needed to organize the FASD material I'd brought to distribute and be on the lookout for other people involved in the case. As I was sitting on a chair in the hallway, I spotted Natalia and Max walking in. Subtly waving to try to get their attention, they came over to me.

"Hi, Mom. Are you trying to get my baby away from us, too?"

I got up and reached out to hug her.

"No, Natalia. I'm here to help you."

We hugged as Max looked on. Knowing Max's troubled past, being in foster care himself, adopted in his teen years, then leaving home, my heart went out to him. I gave him a reluctant but reassuring smile that I was there to help.

"Mom, who is that man with Pop?"

"You'll have to ask Pop. Natalia, I wish you had called me when the baby was born. I've been searching for both of you. I finally got hold of foster care, and they told me you'd be here in court today. What are they advising you to do?"

"A bunch of things . . . we are trying. We have a family meeting with them in the room down the hallway before we go to court. They've set up parenting classes and—"

Max jumped in. "Anger management classes for me. I know I have problems, I really do, but I don't know how to fix it."

"Mom, Max is not evil. He is trying. We both are."

At that moment, some of the foster care case workers in the hallway prompted Natalia and Max to come to the family meeting.

"Mom, we have to go to the meeting. Why don't you come? I think it would help us."

"Natalia, I don't know if I'm allowed. You go and I'll catch up with you after I talk to them. Go, they're calling you."

As Natalia and Max walked to the meeting room, the caseworker called out loudly, looking for the baby's maternal grandparents.

A voice from down the hall responded. Quickly gathering my FASD materials, I headed over to the caseworker to introduce myself, and I saw Natalia's dad introduce his girlfriend as the grandmother.

Looking at him, I said, "Well, I guess congratulations are in order if you're now married. I was of the understanding that as of last week you were still single."

One of the social workers took me aside and whispered in my ear. "I see what's going on here; you are the maternal grandmother, right?"

"Yes, I am."

"We need to talk later."

"Okay, and I have some information to give you so you have a better understanding of Natalia."

"Okay, let's do that. You should be in the family meeting, if the parents agree. Let me go talk to them and I'll be right out."

She went into the room only to come right back out.

"Your daughter would like you in the meeting, but Max said it was only for them. He's a handful, isn't he?"

"Yes, he is. It's okay. I'll wait and we'll talk later." I handed her the information about FASD.

In the meantime, I tried to recollect who Natalia had been talking to in the hallway. Making my way to the other people I believed were involved in the case, I introduced myself and handed out FASD literature to Max's attorney, Natalia's attorney, several foster care caseworkers, and anyone else that might benefit from the information. As I was doing this, I noticed a woman walking in my direction. Dressed in a business suit, she stood out from the crowd, and she seemed to walk with purpose, not glancing at the others in the hallway who might have been obstructing her path. I figured she had to be important and introduced myself.

"Hi, I'm Natalia's mom, and she's here for the deprivation trial or review of her baby. Are you familiar with this case?"

As the woman looked straight through me, it was obvious she was uncomfortable with my question. It was the only time I felt I'd encountered someone who wasn't interested in something that might help Natalia or, for that matter, the baby.

"Yes, I'm familiar with the case."

She didn't tell me her connection to it and she wasn't going to.

"I have some information about Natalia's disability that might be helpful to you in understanding her behaviors. Natalia is a good, loving person—"

She cut me off with a curt, "Thanks, you already gave me information."

She wasn't interested in what I had to say and didn't take the materials I was offering.

As I've learned through the years, FASD caregivers have

limited energy to expend. Don't waste it on someone who isn't open to listen and learn. It's not worth it, and it will only lead to exhaustion. I moved on to someone else who might be more receptive to learning about the underlying cause of all this dysfunction: FASD. The caseworkers from foster care that day were great. They accepted the informational materials and were tirelessly trying to assist Natalia and Max. Where were they when I made the phone calls to their offices months ago? Thank God they were available now!

Natalia and Max came out of the meeting, and Max walked up to me.

"Natalia's mom, can I talk to you for a minute?"

I stepped back. The smell of homelessness and cigarettes was overwhelming. People with FASD sometimes lack personal hygiene skills, especially when they're living on the street. It was becoming more apparent to me that Max might also be on the FASD spectrum. Nevertheless, I realized this was not the time to detach from hearing what he had to say, so I kept my distance and listened.

"Yes, Max, and please just call me Ms. Jacobus or Melissa, whatever you and Natalia are comfortable with."

"Okay, Ms. Jacobus. Uh, these papers were left on the table in the family meeting room. I read through them, and they look like they could be written about me. Natalia said that she has a disability. Well, I think I have that same disability, just a little different than Natalia's."

Good Lord . . . I mean, really, the Lord is good! Max gets it.

"Natalia has told me before that you've tried to help her, and you've spoken to the governor about this," Max said. "Thank you for the work you are doing. Do you think they will ever help people like us?"

"I'm working on it, Max. Now, if you and Natalia want to rejoin your daughter, you have to do what foster care tells you to do. Attend court, go to visitations to see her, and take the classes that they are requiring."

Natalia and Max nodded that they understood.

And since I was on a roll, I said, "Use the services that they are giving you, be respectful, and don't hang out with the wrong people." Knowing they might need clarification, I added, "Which means people who will get you into trouble. Use good judgment, no drugs, do pray, and don't smoke, it's not good for you!"

Natalia nodded to me as she rubbed Max's back. At this point, he was looking down but not rudely ignoring me, as it could be interpreted.

Trying to cram all this information into their thought processes probably wasn't a good idea, as it was overwhelming. Keeping it short and to the point would have been better, though I convinced myself if they got half of what I said, then it was okay for me to say it. Not necessarily the best way to look at it, though it was well-intended. Still, as receptive language or processing information can be extremely difficult to comprehend and stressful, and they were about to experience much more of it in the courtroom, they didn't need the deluge I just threw at them. I knew better and should have taken that into consideration. When their anxiety levels increase, their coping behaviors can be misinterpreted unfairly. Trying to make amends, I gave them a warm, reassuring smile and told them they were doing the right thing by being present at court.

As the courtroom doors were opening and everyone was being corralled in, I reached into my pocket and felt the prayer items I had brought for Natalia, in case she was at court and I ran into her. I'd forgotten that I'd brought them and wasn't sure if I would see her after court. I quickly pulled them out, giving one to her and one to Max. Natalia hugged me, and as she did, Max reached out to me to do the same. I looked at him, said a quick prayer of *God help him*, and gave his arm a gentle squeeze.

Natalia's dad walked by, saying under his breath, "Disgusting, I can't believe this." Understanding his disgust but not his disdain, I ignored it and walked into the courtroom.

What happened next in the juvenile court for the deprivation trial was unimaginable. Natalia had an attorney, Max had an attorney, Natalia's dad had an attorney, foster care was present, and the baby had two women representing her. One was an attorney, and the other was the woman who shunned me in the hallway. She was the baby's guardian ad litem, a special representative appointed by the court.

During the court proceedings everyone had their say, except me, as I sat in the gallery, biting my tongue. It was difficult not to jump out of my seat as I watched DS's attorney walk around with the information I had supplied to DS months earlier, in the hopes it might enable the hospital staff to help Natalia and the baby. I had done all the work of gathering this information over the past fifteen years, yet it seemed that he was given all the credit. I could only sit there and pray for God-given strength to keep me from grabbing the papers from his attorney's hands and cross-examining Natalia's dad about how he had gathered the information and an explanation of what it all meant.

Since the baby was placed in foster care, foster care's goal was to reunite Natalia with her baby, under their guidance. Her dad's request to take temporary placement of the baby was rejected by family and children services, due to Natalia's poor relationship with him and the possibility she wouldn't visit the baby if she was placed with him. Because he'd dropped Natalia off at a motel when she was eight months pregnant and told me he was done with her, I was confused by his request and the fact he was even there. My head was spinning.

The courtroom was adjourned, and we were all sent back into the hallway. Natalia's attorney, whom I had not yet met, pulled me aside and asked to talk to me privately.

As I walked into a private conference room with her, I looked for Natalia, but she was already gone.

"Natalia has said a few things to me that I need to clarify," the attorney said.

"How can I help?"

"Why does her dad want this baby and why isn't Natalia in agreement?"

160

"I don't know why he would try to take custody of the baby. However, it's Natalia's decision, and her decision should be respected."

The attorney nodded, understanding.

I shared some of my experiences in raising Natalia, along with my concerns. Then I gave her the paperwork on Natalia's diagnosis of ND-PAE (FASD). Thankfully, the attorney's prior career had been in education, and she understood developmental and intellectual disabilities.

"Are you interested in taking custody of the baby?"

"Natalia and I have had many talks about her coming home with me, and I would help her care for the baby, but Natalia is her mom. We spoke while she was in jail, and when she got out, before the baby was born, Natalia thought she could do this on her own and didn't want my help, as there would be boundaries at home," I said. "But now that she's under the guidance of foster care, and they're helping her get back on her feet and helping Max with his issues, she might be more inclined to accept help."

"So why did you come to the hearing?" she asked.

"There are so many individuals who are trying to make a decision on Natalia's behalf. I wanted to educate them so they gained a better understanding of her disability and how to help her. Natalia has missed court dates and visitation. Not because she didn't want to be there, but because her executive functions are impaired; in this case, time management. If court was first thing in the morning, she most likely would have trouble arriving on time. So many factors are playing out here that appear to be willful actions but are actually the secondary challenges of FASD."

"Is she capable of caring for the baby?"

"With the proper guidance, support, and interventions, Natalia could care for her. This is the reason I'm distributing the FASD information, trying to educate everyone involved in this case so Natalia gets every available opportunity to take care of her. Again, with supportive housing, parenting classes, and an understanding of her disability, it could work. She is kind and loving and should have every right to be understood. She needs help navigating through life. She doesn't need help teaching her how to love. Her mother's love for her baby is undeniable."

"This must be very difficult to go through as you try to help her," she said. "Here's my card. Feel free to get in touch with me and I'll help as much as I can."

I thanked her and we left the room, going our separate ways.

The decision on who would care for Natalia's daughter was Natalia's, not mine. I was there to support her in every way possible, especially if it was to provide greater insight into Natalia's behavior to those assisting her. I would do it. A mother's love is undeniable, and I loved Natalia.

But at the end of the day, it was Natalia's call.

Chapter 24

Calling for Help

Waking up to a familiar sound, I checked my alarm clock but didn't remember setting it. Dazed, I realized it was my cell phone, and it was across the bedroom on my desk. I ran to answer the call, wondering if it was the police, hospital, or maybe a wrong number. I grabbed the phone and heard Natalia's voice on the other end.

"Hi, Mom. Were you sleeping?"

"Well, yes, but it's okay. How and where are you, and what time is it?"

"It's around five in the morning. I'm at a park in North Atlanta. I need help. I don't know what to do."

"Are you alone? Or is Max with you?"

"Max is with me. Can you come help us?"

"Yes. Tell me where you are."

"Well, I don't really know, some park. Let me put Max on the phone."

Max immediately got on the phone, his uninhibited confidence and charm in full force.

"Hello, Ms. Jacobus. How are you this morning? Your daughter Natalia and I certainly appreciate your time coming to help us."

I could tell Max was trying to be charming, but I wasn't in the mood to be schmoozed. He was morphing into the person he figured would benefit him the most. Still, he was being respectful and I should have been thankful, but I was guarded. At this point, if it benefited him, which in turn benefited Natalia, I was all in.

"Max, just tell me where you are, and I'll come help you."

Max told me where they were in North Atlanta. He'd lived there after he was adopted and because he was familiar with the area, he had come back there to find a job. Of course, Natalia and Max had no money and wanted help paying for a hotel so they could use it as a home base while he was on his job search.

I felt I couldn't go at this alone as I knew Max's behavior could be erratic. I was concerned with who else they might be hanging out with. I needed to call in reinforcements. Since the SWAT team wasn't available, the next best thing was Diane! I called her and explained the situation, though an explanation wasn't needed. As soon as she heard my voice at that early hour, she knew something was up. She came to my house and off we went into the uncharted waters that awaited us.

Natalia and Max were at a café just inside a Target store. They looked tired and needed showers, though they were okay. As Diane and I planned our strategy, we knew we needed to divide and conquer. Natalia would go with me to get groceries and talk. Diane would talk to Max, keeping him occupied.

As Natalia and I walked around the store getting groceries, she mentioned Max's obsession with peanut butter. We made sure he got his peanut butter along with the items I would purchase. It was evident there was a backstory about peanut butter, which I would most likely hear about later. In the meantime, peanut butter was going to be the carrot on the stick that could help lead Max in the right direction. Walking down the various aisles we passed by the infant items. Seeing those prompted Natalia into a conversation about not being able to care for the baby. She told me she wanted her daughter out of foster care and was adamant that she wanted to choose her baby's adoptive parents.

This was the first time she'd given me a definitive decision about the baby's future. I had offered Natalia the opportunity to come home, and I would help her with the baby. She didn't want to come home and would rather stay on the street with Max. She said she was devoted to Max, and she was going to stand by her man, even though running from her man would have been a better choice. No chance of that happening.

Making our way back to the table where we'd left Max and his new best friend Diane, it was evident Diane had worked her magic, making him feel comfortable enough to trust her. Max's moods were very delicate. He had to be handled very carefully, as his behavior was reactionary with explosive outbursts. He had great difficulty processing information, which seemed to frustrate him further.

He couldn't see the reality of their living situation. Fortunately, Natalia could, which helped steer them toward a livable path. They had problems with judgment, choices, and understanding consequences of their behaviors. They were naïve, and trusted people who were not good influences. But as odd as it was, Natalia and Max's relationship worked for them . . . for now. I didn't know Max's heart, but I did know Natalia's, and Max was imbedded in hers. I wondered if Natalia felt a sense of responsibility to him. I didn't know why she was committed to him. She has an incredibly loving heart, even if it was misguided.

Diane and I glanced at each other, knowing we needed to strategize on our next move, and excused ourselves. We told them we were going to drive around and look for a hotel that I could afford for them to stay in for a few days. They could relax at the table in the Target café, eating the food we had just purchased. We let them know we'd be right back, but I think both of us wanted to get in the car and drive far, far away. Reaching out to help someone up close and personal can be frightening when they have experienced sleep deprivation and lack of nutrition, which can alter their mood. When Diane and I were in South Atlanta watching them on security video with the SWAT team standing guard, we were physically safe. However, the situation here felt volatile.

As we got in my car, we discussed the options. We were unsure what Max might do next. Natalia was the main priority, as was her baby. We realized these two needed a place to stay, and for the love of God, they needed a shower. Diane and I agreed that getting them into a hotel for a few days, trying to find a clinic to check on Natalia's medical needs, and getting them to social services for food stamps and some type of assisted living arrangements was essential. As we drove around, we soon found a hotel. We went in and spoke to the manager, explaining Natalia's and Max's situation. And then I saw the sign hanging on the wall—like manna from heaven—the hotel would supply toiletries, such as toothbrushes and toothpaste. These kids not only needed showers, they needed to brush their teeth.

Fortunately, they still had teeth! Immediately, I paid for three nights, which made me responsible for any damage to the room while they were there. No drugs, no smoking. Certainly, Max could hold off from smoking in the room.

While Diane and I drove back to the Target, we stalled as long as we could, trying to figure out how we were going to safely pull off helping them. For our own safety, we also knew we needed to know what was in the backpack they took everywhere, which could contain anything from drugs to weapons. We had been gone longer than we had intended. Natalia knew I was a bit directionally challenged and had called several times to ask if we were okay. Using that to my advantage, I told Natalia that we were trying to find our way back to the Target. She put Max on the phone, who guided us back, giving him confidence and validation that we trusted him. In turn, I hoped he would trust us as their life coaches for the next couple of days.

When we returned to the café where we'd left them, we could feel the glares and stares from others who were sipping their morning coffee. We understood. The situation was odd, and who knows what conversations had taken place while we were gone. There seemed to be a men's prayer group gathering, perhaps they were aware of Natalia's and Max's situation, and were praying for them or us, realizing we were trying to help them. We'd take it!

Telling them we'd found a hotel down the street, we walked to our car and explained that before we all got in the car, we were going to check their backpack. Perhaps because they were shocked, or possibly relieved, that we were helping them, Max opened the backpack, and we went through their possessions: vitamins, Natalia's important papers (good girl), a few granola bars, and there it was—a pellet gun, which looked like a revolver with an orange-tipped muzzle. They said they carried it for their safety. We told them it could be mistaken for a real gun, and they could get hurt if a police officer or someone else felt threatened by it. We convinced Max to let us sell it at a pawnshop, and we would give him the money. Placing the pellet gun in the back of the car, far from his reach, we were off to the hotel, which would be their home for a few days.

When we dropped them off, we told them to get plenty of rest, shower, and be ready early the next morning as we would take them to apply for jobs, go to social services for financial assistance, and take Natalia to a clinic to check her medical needs. Having us schedule and navigate these appointments would ensure they would keep them. They thanked us and we left the hotel.

On the way home, Diane said she would be ready in the morning with whatever I needed. I knew the first order of business was to spray down my back seat with Lysol, as the smell was pretty bad, and God knows what germs they were carrying—those could have been more destructive than the pellet gun.

My work that evening was to call the adoption attorney I had hired when I adopted my children. It had been years since I'd spoken with her, and I wasn't sure if she was still practicing. I needed her advice with Natalia's situation. Ironically, her office was a short distance from the hotel where Natalia and Max were staying. Another order of business that evening was to find a family clinic for Natalia and a shelter that might be able to assist them beyond the three days in the hotel.

It was going to be a long night of research, but it would be a longer day tomorrow to put it all into action.

I prayed Natalia and Max would take showers; it would be hard to stomach their smell in a confined car all day. Car windows would be rolled down if that was the case. Good hygiene habits can be a challenge for those with FASD. Many end up on the street for days and weeks and months and don't realize they need to shower so that the people who are trying to help them can be comfortable in close proximity. Although we may think that the prospect of a refreshing shower would help get them off the street, nope, their minds don't work that way due to limited self-awareness. And brushing their teeth? That's not on their radar, either.

Brushing my teeth before turning in, I reflected on how thankful I was to see Natalia again. She was alive and well. Morning would come soon, and I needed to be well-rested to survive the day ahead, although I wasn't entirely sure if they would still be at the hotel when Diane and I arrived in the morning.

Falling asleep in prayer, I placed everything in God's hands, again.

Chapter 25

The Australian Bakery

Diane arrived bright and early at my house, ready for whatever was in store for us. As we made the hour's drive in typical Atlanta traffic to the kids' hotel, we discussed the priorities for the day. Number one, of course, was making sure they were still at the hotel. Number two was making sure they had showered, and number three was making sure they had brushed their teeth.

The men's shelter's intake was at a specific time in the morning, and we needed to be there to reserve Max's spot and check on an affiliation with a women's shelter. Next stop on the schedule would be the family health center clinic for Natalia, then the nearby Georgia Department of Human Services to look into further financial assistance and for possible jobs in the area.

Thinking about the day's events, I dreaded dealing with a few of those so-called professionals who work with people with mental disorders, but who don't "get it." For example, taking Natalia to receive help when she seems capable of speaking for herself can be extremely difficult. On one occasion, despite my coaching her prior to meeting with the "resource professional," Natalia hit a stumbling block and couldn't adequately express what she needed. She looked to me for help, telling the woman that she had a disability, I was her mother, and she needed me to speak on her behalf. The woman, belittling Natalia, told her she didn't look like she had a disability, and she wouldn't allow me to help. Here's how that conversation went:

"Well, honey, how old are you?"

"I'm twenty," Natalia said.

"Well, are you going to have Mommy helping you when you turn twenty-one?"

I jumped in. "So, how old are you?"

"Thirty-five," she said.

"Oh, I see you are wearing glasses. Are you going to take those glasses off when you turn thirty-six?"

The woman called her supervisor, telling the supervisor to come to the front desk immediately, as she was dealing with a very rude person—me!

I thanked her and took my seat with Natalia.

While we were waiting for the supervisor, Natalia said something very thoughtful about her challenges.

"Mom, things are hard for me. I need assistance just to get the assistance. I'm sorry that woman was rude to you. It's not right."

"I know, Natalia. I'd say that woman has her own disability of not understanding."

As I recalled that encounter, I could only hope we wouldn't face the same discrimination we experienced that day.

Arriving at the hotel around 8:00 a.m., Diane and I realized we might miss the window of opportunity at the men's shelter. When I spoke with the shelter the day before, they explained there was a morning intake to place a name on the list for evening entry. In the late afternoon, that person had to go back to secure their place for the evening. The shelter doesn't let anyone hang out there for the day, as they want to encourage the men to work during the day and return at night.

Working around the shelter's schedule was probably the least of our challenges. Getting Max and Natalia out the door to make these appointments would be the greater challenge.

Certainly, they would be up and ready to go!

As I knocked on the door to the hotel room, there was no answer. Boy, I might have spoken too soon.

"Natalia, good morning. It's Mom."

No answer.

"Natalia, good morning, it's Mom. Please open the door, it's time to go."

No answer.

"Natalia, I hope you are awake. It's Mom, and it's time to go."

No answer.

Knocking very loudly now—

"Natalia, please open the door. I've paid for the room and have the ability to get the manager to open the door for me."

Max answered.

"Yes, we are up, but we're in the shower."

At this point, Diane glanced at me as if to say, "Melissa, I got this one."

She stepped up to the door and began to knock even louder. We couldn't believe Max's nonsense about them being in the shower.

"Max, you heard Ms. Jacobus. Now open the door."

"Hello, Natalia's mom's friend. We are in the shower."

As there was no sound of running water, Diane fired back. "Max, if the water's not running, you can't call it a shower. Now open the door or we will open it with the manager present."

Yes, sirree, there was a reason I brought her along.

Max opened the door, fully dressed in the same clothing and smell as the day before.

"Oh, hello, Natalia's mother and Natalia's mother's friend."

For some reason, Max could not grasp Diane's name, Ms. Preedy.

"Max, call her 'Ms. Pretty,' like the word 'pretty' in 'she looks pretty.'"

Because he had difficulty responding with typical social cues, I thought using some humor might jolt him into focusing on the matter at hand—getting ready and out the door, rather than getting angry because he wasn't ready for the day's appointments. They were going to these appointments, frustrated or not.

"You two needed to be ready when we arrived," I said. "We have limited time to get to these appointments. We've most likely missed out on the homeless shelter's morning intake and now we'll try to make it to their afternoon one."

Max was grumbling the entire time.

Natalia rubbed his back, whispering to him that I was trying to help him, as she gave me a reassuring look that he would comply.

Diane shook her head, as she knew what we were in for.

Knowing we were on borrowed time with Max's limited attention span and unpredictable behavior, I remembered the food we'd purchased for them the day before.

"Max, grab some of the food I bought you yesterday. You two can eat it in the car while we head out to the family health center to have Natalia checked out."

Fearing I'd given him too many directions and he'd be overwhelmed trying to process them, he surprised me. He grabbed the food and we all got in the car. Diane in the front passenger seat, Natalia and Max in the back seat.

Not only did they get in the car, but that horrible smell got in the car with them.

"Did you take a shower yesterday after we left the hotel?"

"Yes, Mom, we did."

As she spoke, the smell jumped from her breath.

"And what about the toothbrushes that the front desk had for you? Did you go and get them?"

"Oh, no Natalia's mother, we didn't have time to do that."

"So, Max, what you're telling me is that you have not brushed your teeth?"

Deciding not to wait for an answer and the possibility of getting sick from their breath, I reached in my purse for mints I'd picked up at a restaurant some time ago. They were probably as old as the hills, but at least they would keep the air inside the car tolerable until we could get to a convenience store for something stronger.

The family health clinic was the first order of business. As we drove, Max was our tour guide, pointing out various places he had gone with his adoptive parents—restaurants, fencing lessons, church, and an Australian bakery in the town square. It was evident his parents cared for him and his well-being. Taking in a teenager from foster care is not easy. Though limited in scope, the stories he told of his time with them painted a picture of faith and restoration for a boy who didn't have a good start in life. They were good people.

"Hey, Natalia's mom, can we go to the Australian bakery? It's right around the corner from here."

"Max, we need to get to the clinic first to have Natalia examined."

I was fearful she might be pregnant again and not getting proper nutrition for the baby. She had also been having inconsistent and painful periods.

"She doesn't need to go to the doctor. She's healthy. If anyone needs to go it would be me, but I'd rather go to the Australian bakery. My parents loved it and we went all the time. They knew me there."

"Well, Max, Natalia could be pregnant, and I want to make sure she and the baby are healthy."

"Oh, she's not pregnant. I think I'm sterile because she gave me some kind of disease, and I should be the one to get checked out. So let's go to the Australian bakery."

"Max, if we have time at the end of the day, I'll take you there. It sounds like your parents were really good people from all the things you're telling me you did with them."

"They were okay, but my mom was mean. She wouldn't let me eat peanut butter."

Okay, I knew there was a story there.

"What's the deal with the peanut butter, Max?"

"She said a couple of tablespoons was a serving size and that was all I could eat."

At this point I could guess what probably had happened. Max hoarded peanut butter, eating container after container of it, could have gotten sick, and his mother had to limit the amount he could have. She most likely reasoned with him about a serving-size portion, which he couldn't comprehend.

"Well Max, if you ate jars of it, which is what could have happened, you might have gotten a stomachache, and I bet your mom didn't want you to feel bad. She sounds like a nice, smart person who cared about you. I would have done the same thing."

"Well when she did it, I showed her. I took my money and went and bought a bag of chocolate candy. Ate the whole bag of it. She was really mad then!"

And Max you probably got a really bad stomachache, so I guess you really showed you.

And just in the nick of time, before he could share any more of the story, we drove up to the family clinic. It would open in about a half hour. Max, of course, insisted that gave us enough time to go to the Australian bakery.

As we stood outside, waiting for the clinic to open, Max and Natalia told us about their adventures on the street, and his history of foster homes, group homes, and his adoptive parents. He had so much potential for happiness and success, though the system had failed him. It was possible he hadn't been diagnosed correctly, and he knew it. As challenging as he was, there was an inkling of compassion and smarts about him. It was just all cloaked by his disability—neurotransmitters constantly misfiring, creating a personality that was difficult to digest due to his oppositional behavior and limited ability to reason. How could this kid not have found big trouble before now? I knew he couldn't be blamed; his FASD was the cause of most of his problems. And boy, it was almost impossible to give him that out. But as he told me about his challenges, my heart softened to help this young man. He was a survivor, hooked up with Natalia, who was like his life coach, God help them both. Unfortunately, she would continue to ride out his storms to lead him to calmer waters.

To help Natalia, I had to help Max.

Finally, the clinic door opened, and we were allowed in.

"Natalia, go to the front desk and tell them what you need."

"Okay, Mom, and what do I need?"

What she needed was a continuous advocate. Not just a helicopter parent, but the militia with all the protective armor.

Though I was always trying to coach her to help herself, we had time constraints and I stepped in.

"Hi, my daughter is homeless without financial means and needs to be examined for possible pregnancy, STD testing, and anemia. Can you help her?"

"Well, let me see her waiver showing she has no income so I can reduce her financial responsibility."

What? That's the first I had heard of this!

"What is the waiver, and where is she supposed to get it?"

"She needs to go to the department of labor, fill out a form with her Social Security number, and they can check to see if she's employed or not. Bring the waiver back to us and we will get her in to see a doctor."

Oh, okay . . . my daughter, homeless, without transportation of her own, can just ride right over to the department of labor, wait in what is probably a long line, fill out forms to show she has no income, then swing right back over here while you're still open. And maybe she can also swing by the Australian bakery for a few pastries while she's out for the lovely drive around town.

I'd done my research the night before and nowhere did I find this information. Furthermore, the hours of operation listed for the clinic were wrong. So, unless I drive to these places and meet the people in person, I never know what information is correct. I don't have a disability, but after what was going to be an even longer day, I would definitely be impaired!

I was prepared to pay for the cost of the clinic, but I also knew Natalia would be on her own again, and if she needed medical attention, she would need this waiver to help defray the cost.

"Will you please provide me with their address and phone number? And what time is your last appointment?"

With that we were out the door, in the car, and on our way to the department of labor. Of course, Max pointed out if we took his "shortcut," we could go by that darn Australian bakery.

If we did, I would be sure to leave him there!

There was a long line of people waiting for assistance at the department of labor. Because Natalia had a copy of her Social Security card and a few other copies of records I had her keep with her, she got in a shorter line. God help those other people without proper identification. I stood behind her as she applied for the waiver, giving her instructions on what to ask for. Perhaps it might have been a rarity for the clerk behind the desk to see parents like me trying to support their kids, as the clerk helped Natalia promptly, with compassion and efficiency, though possibly out of pity.

We headed back to the family health clinic. Diane told Max to keep his comments about the bakery to himself. I don't believe either one of us could withstand his continued nonsense as we were pressed for time.

The clinic had a few people waiting to be seen and Natalia was next. She went into the examining room alone. Max went outside, as he couldn't sit still. The solitude gave Diane and me some time to talk about the rest of the afternoon.

"Melissa, you're a better person than I am. I've just about had enough of Max."

Diane had kept Max occupied at the café the previous morning, and anytime I needed to talk to Natalia privately, Diane was my wingman, taking bullets intended for me.

"No, Diane, I'm not a better person. I've just had more experience tolerating this type of behavior. I ignore it, maneuver around his challenges, and try to find the window of opportunity to get him from point A to point B so I can help Natalia. Please feel free to say whatever you want when he gets out of hand. I'm just so tired. I don't have the energy to combat him and it wouldn't help anyway."

Diane followed Max outside to keep an eye on him while Natalia was in the examining room. We certainly didn't need him finding trouble outside the clinic. Plus, it was a good opportunity for me to talk with the front desk clerk about Natalia's future care and her financial responsibilities to the clinic. I showed them her passport because they'd questioned her identity. I then showed them my ID, said I was her mother, and would pay for the day's fees.

At this point they were very helpful, understanding the

situation and potential problems Natalia could have in her immediate future. They began to see her life differently than when she first walked in. God knows who comes through that door and those who can't advocate for themselves. I thanked the ladies and gave them my FASD parent advocate contact card, hoping that having two more people who now understood FASD might help the next person with FASD that entered the clinic.

"Mom, I'm done."

"Are you okay?"

"Yes, not pregnant, no STDs like Max said, but I have to go to the drugstore for my birth control medicine."

Natalia and I discussed birth control to prevent additional pregnancies. Though I've never been a proponent of alternatives to natural family planning, I had a realistic view of her challenges and wanted to support her decisions. We'd been fortunate that her baby was born healthy, but we both were concerned about another pregnancy and abortion was never an option. After praying about it, we agreed that a prescription birth control method was the safest and most effective choice. Because she wouldn't remember to take a daily pill, she'd get the birth control shot.

I asked the nurse who was in the waiting area, "We have to go to the drugstore for her birth control prescription and bring it back? They don't keep them here?"

"Yes, that's right, and you will have to hurry because we close in less than an hour."

Immediately, we all got in the car and proceeded to the

closest drugstore, prescription in hand. Walking quickly down the aisle to get to the pharmacist, we knew the clinic might be closed by the time we returned.

As I was paying for the medicine, the clerk asked if I wanted cash back. Max jumped in, asking me to pay for some items he wanted. Diane had already tried to head Max off at the pass, but he was able to slip his request in.

"Max, Ms. Jacobus is taking care of Natalia's medical care, along with helping pay for your hotel, food, and driving you all around."

"Well, I just thought since she was paying for something else, and she was getting cash back . . . she wouldn't mind . . . uh—"

"Max, Ms. Jacobus is not an ATM machine!"

Max was silent, and perhaps he understood her point. I know I did, and again, I was so thankful to have her support, and her wit. She was strong, direct, and darn right funny.

The clinic was still open. They administered Natalia's shot, and we were off to the men's shelter for the afternoon intake.

We missed their deadline and were told to come back early the next morning for the next intake, which is what we planned to do. It was late in the afternoon, and I mentioned that Diane's dog, Zoey, needed to be taken out, as we had been gone all day, and we had over an hour's drive home.

As we headed back to the hotel, Max brought up the

Australian bakery again, which, at this time of the day, was likely closed.

"So, since we are done with our errands, do you think we can go to the Australian bakery before going to the hotel?"

"Max, as I said a minute ago, Ms. Preedy and I need to get back home so she can take her dog out. We've got a long drive back in traffic, so no, we won't have time to go to the Australian bakery today."

Diane and I looked at each other, wondering if Max was going to react or say a simple "okay."

Instead, Max piped up from the back seat. "Figures!"

Although his answer was almost comical, the fact his emotional inability to relate to the priorities of the day rested on whether he would get to go to the Australian bakery was sad.

Tomorrow would be another busy, long day—homeless shelter and possible job search.

And if things went smoothly, maybe we'd be able to drop by that Australian bakery.

Chapter 26

Plan B

After getting up early, packing up any clothes I could find for Natalia to wear and rummaging through my St. Vincent de Paul box for the needy to supply clothes to the homeless men's shelter, I left the house to pick up Diane, who lived a few blocks away. Driving the short distance to Diane's house, there was no shortage of mental anguish swirling around in my mind, wondering what was waiting for Diane and me when we arrived at the hotel.

Despite a good night's sleep, I had woken up with the same worrisome thoughts I had when I went to bed. Now I needed to purge them from my mind. Would Natalia and Max be ready to go to the men's shelter for intake? Would there be a caseworker available to help them? What about Natalia's daughter? Natalia wanted her safe, wanted to find a home with parents she would select. How in the world could this be accomplished when I didn't even know if they would be at the hotel when Diane and I arrived?

Diane and I discussed the multitude of these all-consuming concerns during the hour-long drive in rush hour traffic. We arrived at the hotel at 7:30 a.m., knowing we needed to be at the homeless shelter soon thereafter. The manager looked at me with concern as we walked past the registration desk. Diane and I had the feeling Natalia and Max might soon be on the move, as the day before Max had indicated things were not going as he had planned. He was impulsive, could be explosive, and it was evident he wasn't processing information well enough to understand we could—and were—helping him. We knew we were on limited time. Natalia's health and her baby's future could be determined in the next couple of hours, and we would do our best to maneuver through the chaos that would like-ly unfold.

"Natalia and Max, we're here. It's time to go."

Max opened the door. He was not happy to see us and obviously not prepared for the day. The room was a mess. Cigarette butts on the floor. Smoking was not allowed, and I knew there was a possibility I would be paying a hefty fine because of their carelessness.

"Max, I hope you didn't smoke in this room. I'm respon-sible for the payment and additional charges if you did. Please help me pick things up."

Max glared at me and headed out the door. Diane fol-lowed behind him, telling him he needed to respect and appreciate what we were trying to do for him.

"Mom, I'll pick things up."

"Natalia, it's not your job to pick up after Max. He needs to take ownership of his behavior. Natalia, we've got a lot to do today. Is Max going to be okay?"

"He didn't sleep much because he went out last night and isn't in a good mood."

Good God, what does that mean? Is he on something? Is he manic? Could he be carrying drugs with him now?

"Natalia, we need to get going."

At that moment she went over to the sink and began brushing her teeth. I wasn't about to stop her since, presently, this was a rare occurrence. But I knew this was my chance to talk with her about coming home, and she'd have to listen while she was bent over the sink with a toothbrush in her mouth.

"Natalia, Max was out all night? It's obvious that he isn't capable to care for you or your daughter. Just come home with me. Let's get her and I'll help you with her. You can meet up with Max later, after he gets his life together."

"Mom, Max needs me. He can't do it on his own."

"Natalia, Max can't stay out of his own way. He's going to bring harm to the both of you. Can't you see he's not making sense right now?"

As she spit blood into the sink, she looked up at me and said, "He makes sense to me, Mom."

I knew she wasn't coming home. And she wasn't making sense. She had not yet hit bottom in her existence with Max. Until that time, there was no talking any sense into her.

"Well, let's get your things out of the room. You won't be able to stay here any longer because you're not respectful of the hotel's policy."

We walked out of the room and to the registration desk. I asked the manager to settle our bill, saying the kids would be checking out.

Outside in the parking lot, Max was sitting on the curb, smoking a cigarette. Diane was trying to explain the plans for the day, and he obviously didn't want to hear them. Natalia and I were now within earshot, and I could see and hear that Max was overwhelmed.

"Max, we need to get you to the men's shelter," Diane said. "They'll help you find work and a more permanent place to live."

"We're not going to the shelter! Ms. Jacobus's plan didn't work."

"What do you mean Ms. Jacobus's plan didn't work? She's trying to help you find a place to live and a job."

"Ms. Jacobus's Plan A didn't work, so we're on to Plan B."

Diane, in her quick-witted way, shot back at Max. "So, Max, what's Plan B? Sitting on the curb?"

Natalia began rubbing his back, trying to calm him down. He was not cooperating and began raising his voice and waving his arms. He got up, grabbed the ripped, shoestring-tied backpack from the curb, and handed it to Natalia.

Disgusted with what I was seeing I said, "Natalia, why are you carrying the backpack?"

"Max has back problems. He can't carry it because it's too heavy. It's fine, Mom. I always carry it."

"Natalia, remember what we talked about while you were brushing your teeth? The offer still stands."

With that, they began walking away from the hotel, down the side of the street toward a shopping center.

I shouted to them, "God be with you."

Wondering what had just happened, Diane and I got in the car to drive home. Although I realized how quickly things had gone downhill, I thought maybe we could turn them around just as quickly before Natalia and Max were too far from our reach. We pulled into a parking lot and prayed, asking God for His Grace and the presence of mind to know how to help them.

"God, please help us help these kids, give us patience of mind and guidance on what to do."

After our prayer, I felt led to call the family adoption attorney that I had contacted a few days ago for advice. I knew it was probably too early for her to be in the office, and it would be God's hands if she were to answer.

"Hello?"

Caught off guard, I must have sounded frantic and pathetic.

"Hi, this is Melissa. Are you available to talk with Natalia and Max about their options if someone is ready to adopt their baby? I wish I had the time to fill you in on what just happened this morning at the hotel with them, but I don't."

"Melissa, you will have to bring them to me."

"Okay. Natalia told me she wants to select parents for an adoption. Let me see if we can find them. I'll call you if we do and bring them to you. What's your address?"

I wrote down the address and ended the call. Diane and I knew God's hand was in that phone call. With tears in our eyes and faith filling our hearts, we found strength. I called their cell phone.

"Well, hello, Ms. Jacobus. Can I help you?"

"Hi, Max. I am so sorry about how things transpired at the hotel. I know you and Natalia must be pretty tired and frustrated. I know Ms. Preedy and I are. Before I left my house this morning, I grabbed some clothes for the shelter and some for Natalia. Why don't Ms. Preedy and I meet you and Natalia, and you can go through the clothes and take what you want? I think I have some food, too."

"Okay, I guess that would be all right. We are at a Target, just walking up to the front of the store."

It was like I was talking to an entirely different person. That short walk for Max disengaged him from his emotional chaos. He was calmer and seemed reasonable.

"We'll be right there."

I called the adoption attorney and told her we'd found Natalia and Max and hoped to be at her office within the hour.

Driving up to the store, we spotted Natalia and Max, and they greeted us. Relieved that Max was now calm after their walk, I mentioned that his torn backpack wouldn't hold any of the clothes I'd brought with me and offered to buy them a new backpack. He agreed.

We opened the back of the car, and it was like Christmas morning. Their faces lit up when they saw the clothes that were waiting for them. Natalia's eyes teared, and she whispered to me that the underwear I had brought would come in handy as she had none. It had all been lost one of the many times they'd been kicked out from wherever they were living. How long had she been wearing her present and only clothes? They didn't need just one backpack—they'd need two to carry the clothes they were taking. Max would have to share the burden of carrying their belongings.

We went into Target to shop for backpacks. Diane and Max went down one aisle, Natalia and I another. I asked Natalia about her daughter's future, and she told me she wanted to select parents for her and wanted my help. She and Max planned to move out of state, where apparently Max knew a friend they could live with. As I was giving her a few options for a home for the baby, Max overheard the conversation and walked up. He said he supported Natalia. They wanted to pick the parents, and they would appreciate it if I would help them. Gratitude flooded my heart as I realized our parking lot prayers had been answered.

Finally, we found the backpacks. Since I'm not an ATM machine, I said they'd need to choose backpacks that were on sale. They did, and Natalia told Max I always found a deal when shopping. That's how we managed finances in our home—we were smart shoppers, hand-me-downs were a way of life, and nothing was taken for granted.

As we walked up to the cashier to pay for the backpacks, I said a little prayer aloud asking that they would be cheaper than the noted sale price. Max looked at me, rolling his eyes. As the cashier rang them up, she said all school items were on clearance, with an additional fifty percent off!

Natalia looked at Max with a glimmer in her eyes. "See Max, I told you that my Mom's prayers work."

I smiled at her. "There are angels, Natalia. They are all around us."

When we got back to my car, they removed their items from the old backpack, divided up their belongings, and placed those in their new ones. It was definitely better than Christmas morning!

I was so pleased Natalia had her copies of important papers (birth certificate, passport, and Social Security card), and I helped her secure them in her backpack, along with her clothes and some food.

"Mom, what about my daughter? Will you help us find parents for her?"

Natalia looked at Max and he nodded in agreement.

I called the adoption attorney to let her know we were on our way. We were minutes from a moment that would change all our lives forever.

As we drove, Max organized his new backpack and removed the tags.

Silently praying during the short drive to the attorney's office, I wondered if Max truly understood the incredible impact this unselfish decision would have for their daughter and her future adoptive parents. Was he capable of being thankful for the love and guidance he received from his adoptive parents? Or the help he was receiving now with the selection of parents for his daughter? I saw him proudly hold his new shiny backpack. I was about to get my answer because we were pulling up to the building where these important moments would happen.

"Ms. Jacobus, can I tell you something?"

Surprised, I said, "Sure, Max. What is it?"

"That was really nice of you to buy me and Natalia the backpacks and help us these past couple of days. Natalia has told me that you are a pretty good mom, but I got to tell you, you certainly have an unorthodox way of showing it."

"Well, Max, it sounds like you are being appreciative. And if that's the case, you certainly have an unorthodox way of saying thank you, but I'll take it."

Natalia and Max walked into the attorney's office, as Diane and I followed behind.

I knew God's angels would soon be arriving.

Chapter 27

We Choose You

Walking into the adoption attorney's office was like walking into a comfortable hug, warm and inviting, as if we were in someone's family room. The attorney greeted us and asked Diane and me to stay in the large waiting room while she took Natalia and Max in another room for a private conversation about the adoption and their wishes. Happily anticipating what might take place, I sat close to the hallway they'd entered, thinking I might be able to hear a little of the conversation, but when the door shut behind them, there was no chance of that. Diane sat on the other side of the room.

It was a huge relief to have someone else who understood the process for the decision Natalia and Max were making. I was confirming their wishes and supporting their decision to choose adoptive parents who would love and raise their daughter. It was an incredibly unselfish act of love and faith.

While they were gone, Diane and I sat quietly, waiting and praying that all would go smoothly with the selection of the parents and the process needed to solidify their decision. I felt a sense of relief this was out of our hands and now in the hands of God.

A sound caught my attention, and I watched a couple open the front door. As they looked around the room, there was a sense of humility and anticipation about them. They looked to be in their late thirties. Could this be the couple Natalia and Max had selected?

The attorney called out from the other room, saying she would be with them momentarily.

Diane and I glanced at each other, though we didn't need to say a word. Listening to the adoring couple's whispered conversation, it was evident they were the parents Natalia and Max had selected. If they were to raise the baby with the abundant love that was evident between the two of them, she would be well taken care of.

As we sat across from them, trying not to stare, I prayed they would give her the love, safety, and supportive, faith-filled family environment she deserved. And for the love of God, I prayed for Max's heart to understand the importance of the decision he was making. It was evident that Natalia knew.

As the couple waited, excitement and tears glistening in their eyes, I caught their glance.

"It's going to be all right. Everything is going to be just fine." I told them I was Natalia's mom. Diane introduced herself, and we told them we would keep their new family in our prayers.

Just then, the attorney came out into the waiting area with a big smile on her face.

She greeted them and said Natalia and Max were waiting to meet with them.

I could hardly contain myself as they left the room, immediately jumping out of my seat to sit next to Diane so we could compare our emotional notes on what we were feeling and what we saw in this new couple, soon to be parents.

We were on the same page. Diane even commented that Max better be on Plan A with the rest of us!

After what seemed like forever, they all came out of the room, smiling and teary-eyed.

The attorney said, "Melissa, this is the couple Natalia and Max have selected. We've got everything in order, and I'll be in touch if I need anything else."

"Thank you! I'm here for whatever you need."

Everyone hugged as if we were all old friends, and we knew this extended family would be forever bonded.

We walked out to the car to take Natalia and Max to their next stop, the hotel where they'd stayed when Natalia had to check in with her probation officer. Unsure of their future, they would take it one step at a time, and choosing adoptive parents for their baby had been a huge step in the right direction.

Max smiled at me. "Ms. Jacobus, you know I'm feeling really good about what just happened."

"Max, I am, too! That was a wonderful decision you and Natalia made. So, what are your next plans?"

"Well, Ms. Jacobus, I really think I'd like to be an adoption lawyer when I get older. I want to help people with disabilities like us who know they can't take care of their children."

"Max, I think that is a great idea, and you could do it, too! Get on the right path, work hard, pray, and anything is possible. Don't let your disability define you. We all have strengths and gifts. You just have to find yours, safely!"

We all got into the car, and I reached back to touch Natalia on the knee. "Natalia, how are you doing?"

"What do you mean, Mom?"

"I mean, how are you doing? You did a wonderful thing choosing adoptive parents. You gave them the gift of family. I know how thankful I am to be your mom, and what a beautiful gift you are!"

"Thank you, Mom. I love you. This is what we wanted."

Then she rustled around in the back seat and asked Max to pass her some crackers.

They were content and life was good.

Chapter 28

Prayers Answered

It had been several months since Natalia and Max's meeting with the adoption attorney and the adoptive parents. Today, the attorney, adoptive parents, and Diane (as a witness) were at the court hearing. The outcome was now in the judge's and God's hands. I had stayed home, on my knees in prayer, asking that all would go smoothly and the Holy Spirit would guide the judge's decision. When Diane called to tell me the baby had been successfully adopted by the beautiful parents Natalia and Max had selected, I got off my knees.

It was hard to believe only months earlier, I'd been on my knees looking at security footage in a South Atlanta hotel, trying to find Natalia. I remembered having to clean the dust off myself when I got up from that dirty floor. Now, I was getting up and giving thanks my prayers had been answered. Natalia was alive, her baby was safe and in the loving care of the couple Natalia had selected to be her daughter's parents—her call.

Life had taken so many unexpected turns, and now the winding road could straighten out a little, with a clearer path for the future. Please, dear God, no more issues!

The future for the many homeless and incarcerated people with FASD was not going to be as clear. FASD is very real, and those who aren't aware of it need to be educated. Many people with FASD are out there wandering aimlessly, getting into trouble with the law, and not understanding why their choices don't keep them safe from trouble. There are a lot of multi-diagnoses and nowhere to get concrete information about how to help them.

And where was Maurice? That day at the FASD conference when we met Maurice, I promised Nicky we'd find him. He never left my thoughts. We would try, try, try, and then try some more! Unknown to Maurice, we were both committed to him. I felt as though Maurice was lost out there somewhere, and I could only imagine if Nicky were in his place, lost, yet thinking he could take care of himself. People with FASD might seem overly confident about their abilities, even though the judgment center of their navigation system is compromised. It's similar to what Maurice's social worker had told me—Maurice didn't think he needed anyone to help him, didn't want to be a burden. But as she said, he could not do it alone. He needed help. Nicky and I continued to pray for God's guidance to help us find him or, at the very least, keep him safe.

But first things first . . .

A much-deserved nap was in order. I was taking a breather to get some sleep, then going full force the rest of the day. I was determined to expose FASD for what it was and that it didn't define those who were impacted. It was a wrinkle they needed ironed out, and it would wrinkle again, and the help would be available again. In helping those who are impacted by this "invisible disability," I was determined that society's ignorance would no longer be *the accomplice* to the madness of undiagnosed FASD. So much needed to be done with strategizing and organizing FASD training in Atlanta, getting in touch with local resources and my trusted friend, Billy Edwards, public defender for the mental health courts in LA County. He was well-connected and had recruited national presenters for this type of training. The presenters, who were all experts in FASD, were devoting their lives to helping others.

It was a privilege to hear them present and a comfort that they understood the challenges. And speaking of comforting, I needed that comforting nap to put my brain at rest.

"Nicky, I'm going to take a little rest. What are you up to today?"

He didn't answer, which was unlike him. I walked around the house to look for him.

"Nicky, where are you?"

When I walked into the basement, he was sitting on the sofa watching TV, looking up, but in a subtle way, ignoring me. Although I'd been distracted by Natalia's challenges, I'd noticed he hadn't been himself for months. I hadn't been paying enough attention and just told myself he was busy with work.

"I'm fine, Mom. You're busy, and I'll take care of it."

Yes, I was busy all the time. Jumping from one chaotic mess to the next and probably neglecting him or getting frustrated he wasn't following through with his chores. I had a whole lot of navigating to do for my adult children and no time to navigate my own life. He and I had butted heads, and it was a matter of time before we would have a mini-blowup. Thankfully, we usually were able to talk it out, though most recently we hadn't been able to.

"I can tell something has been going on because when I see behaviors at home that aren't right, it usually means something is happening at work. What's going on?"

"They don't know what they are doing. I'm the only one who does any work. They've scheduled me wrong again. I only have fourteen hours for the week, and there's a guy at work who is like a bully to me and makes fun of my frustrations. I told him I had a disability and he said I didn't. He's one of the assistant managers and keeps giving me more to do while I'm there. I can't do it."

"Tell me what happened and we'll talk about it so you can address it with them."

"Mom, you know it's hard for me. I try but have a hard time getting the information right, especially with scheduling my vacation time. They didn't approve it, and I asked for it months ago. What am I going to do? I have an airline ticket to go see Aunt Kim and Uncle Brian. Brian Matthew and I hang out together. That's my time with them. Babushka and I are going. Plus, Babushka and I always help each other through the airport."

"It will be okay. We'll work through it, Nicky. Let me take a twenty-minute nap to rest my brain and when I wake up, we'll put our heads together and figure it out."

Thinking about his frustration, I knew it was overwhelming for him to be working in an environment that was inundated with multitasking. He had difficulty taking multiple directions from the many managers in the various departments. His ability to process information was impaired, so it layered on the frustration—anxiety from trying to do it right and frustration that it wasn't working. What's more, he believed he was right much of the time because his brain was telling him he did what he was supposed to do. But the reality was he might not have followed through correctly. It was almost like his brain was tricking him. He had worked at this grocery store for about seven years and had done an excellent job, though I had to advocate for him about his disability every three to five months when a new manager just didn't get it or had not read his file. It wasn't a matter of retraining Nicky; it was a matter of educating the managers since his disability was "invisible." Being friendly, willing to help, and handsome certainly didn't help his case of what people believe doesn't "look" like a disability. And he worked so darn hard to make it all seem like it was easy for him, which it wasn't.

Socially, he had some really good friends, though boundaries were still set at home with a curfew—especially when he had to be at work early in the morning because sleep deprivation can wreak havoc on the brain, cause memory loss, and increase anxiety. Knowing that he wanted the independence of an adult—and he was a legal adult—I would need to look into supportive housing where he could have his own place, yet live interdependently. I'd been trying to find that place where he would be accommodated and happy, but there was limited time to look and limited places that were a match. He needed to agree on that place, if and once it was found.

With all that had gone on in the past year, he had coasted. I should have seen it coming.

I knew he had a breaking point; I just didn't realize that point was coming so soon.

2015

Chapter 29

When Hell Freezes Over

The Christmas season seemed to arrive without warning, and my youngest daughter, who was in her early twenties and expecting, came home for some family time. Her life had also not been easy that year, and she needed some TLC for herself and her soon-to-be-delivered beautiful baby girl.

At home, she'd get to enjoy our usual traditions of baking Christmas cookies, watching Christmas movies, and dining on sushi for Christmas Eve dinner. On Christmas morning, after attending mass, we'd have cinnamon rolls and quiche for breakfast, then open presents. The highlight was watching Babushka's shih tzu, Mei Ling, tear the gift-wrap from her doggy toy. One year, Mei Ling ripped open the package, only to ignore the toy. She knew it had been re-gifted from the previous year and snubbed her little shih tzu nose at it. Ordinarily, she's enthusiastic in the spotlight, tearing open her gift as we all laugh hilariously. Knowing that next year she'd have to share the spotlight with a beautiful baby girl, we'd made sure she received a new toy.

On Christmas morning, we headed to mass for the eight-thirty service. The pastor of our church was also a gift. As always, we knew he'd share the true meaning of Christmas, and no one ever slept through his homily, as his words were always so insightful. Speaking of sleeping, earlier that morning, my daughter had mentioned that her baby must have been sleeping, as she wasn't feeling her move. As I relayed this information to my mother, she kept a close, prayerful eye on my daughter as we entered the church, and sat next to her. As my daughter, Nicky, and my mother and I stood up for the processional of the priest and altar servers, my mother glanced at her and whispered to me that the baby had dropped.

As the music from the church organ played, my daughter abruptly leaned over to me, saying she could feel her baby moving. As I smiled at my mother, whose strong faith seemed to keep us all spiritually grounded, I was reminded of the biblical passage where Mary greeted Elizabeth "and her baby leaped in her womb." Just then, I remembered my mother's middle name was Elizabeth. My mother always said moments like this are the presence of the Holy Spirit. This all seemed so fitting and what a blessing! And that was not the only blessing that morning. As we were leaving mass, the pastor gave my daughter and her soon-to-be-born baby girl the gift of a special blessing, while I said an extra prayer under my breath. "Deliver this baby . . . now, and safely!"

I added another prayer that evening before bedtime. Getting on those trusted knees, I prayed like the "Charles" Dickens that the baby would be born before my daughter left.

Early the next morning, she came out of her bedroom, complaining of a stomachache. It was my late father's birthday, and my mother and I had planned on attending a morning church service in his memory. When I asked my daughter if her stomach pains were coming in waves, she moaned yes. I figured she was in labor, so we scooped up the hospital overnight bag and a newborn baby outfit she'd received as Christmas gifts and off we went. She was a trouper during labor, but when the midwife suggested she cut the umbilical cord, she looked at me in shock, like she was about to deliver another baby. Seeing her despair, without hesitation, I cut the cord and tied it into a Christmas bow! It was a Christmas miracle! This angel of a baby girl was born.

The months flew by—summer came and went, and we were back to the holiday months with Thanksgiving peeking around the corner. The holidays were a stressful time for Nicky as the grocery store was very hectic during the season. We worked through challenges and made the best of it. Vacation schedules were an issue again, though this time we were a little more prepared. Nicky took his Florida trip to see the relatives, which was a wonderful time for him to re-charge and simply have fun. He and his babushka usually traveled together, which gave them additional grandson-grandmother bonding time. And me, I needed alone time to pick up the pieces still scattered from the previous year.

The year continued to be busy as I traveled to FASD-related speaking engagements in other states to talk with families caring for loved ones with an FASD. The speaking engagements were helpful, as they created a framework for the training that would be organized in Atlanta the coming year. In the meantime, my personal family challenges continued, including concerns for both of my daughters. I didn't know the whereabouts of one, and the other was juggling work, school, and being a new mom. On top of that, my mother's health was declining. All this seemed to hijack any downtime or time to address Nicky's ongoing questionable behavior. I was overwhelmed.

Knowing one thing that would make Nicky's day or, for that matter, his year, would be if his brother came to visit him from the military. My oldest son had been in the service for about four years. During that time, he'd only come home for his sister's high school graduation and on a layover at the airport with his wife. Nicky missed his brother terribly, and whenever we thought we could plan a trip to see him, something else was going on at home that was a priority.

He and his wife had recently had a baby, and a homecoming in Atlanta would give Nicky a chance to spend time with him and give me a chance to welcome his wife and their new baby to the stomping grounds where he grew up.

Nicky, excited for his brother's visit, helped plan what they would do while at home, and we wanted to make sure there were no mishaps or miscommunication in scheduling

Nicky's time off from work. Due to Nicky's challenges, a mishap happened anyway. I needed to plan a trip to the grocery store to talk to his manager.

Preparing for my son's and his family's visit, we tied a yellow ribbon around the oak tree in the front yard. Their homecoming was great—a Braves game, a day at the spa for his wife and me to get to know each other better, traditional board games at the kitchen table, dinner at our favorite neighborhood Mexican restaurant, a home-cooked Russian dinner, and another night of barbecue with family and friends. It was a week to celebrate all our family traditions while spotlighting the joy of having everyone together. Although we missed Natalia, we prayed that next time we'd all be together.

As the week ended, we knew we wouldn't let so much time go by between visits again. They left with a hug and prayer for their safe return. It was wonderful to have spent quality time with them, enjoying their beautiful family. I was relieved and elated at the success he was having in the military and the love he had found with his wife and their precious son. Thankfully, we took lots of photos, which I planned to attach to an email I was sending them, reminiscing about the visit. Unfortunately, the email and pictures would have to wait as there were too many to attach in one email, and I had a trip to prepare for.

The trip was only for a couple of days and only a few hours away. Nicky would be home, looking after Babushka next door, and she would be checking in on him. He seemed a little distant, perhaps feeling neglected, as I said goodbye, though I made sure the refrigerator was stocked, so at least his stomach wouldn't feel neglected. He and I would have some much-needed time together when I returned to talk about whatever was on his mind, which would most likely be his future living arrangements, work changes, and possibly driving soon. He had a sizable savings account I'd coached him to save for his future, and he'd be able to access it soon, under supervision. Although some people with disabilities receive Supplemental Security Income, eligibility is limited, and Nicky's disability didn't yet qualify. I was hoping the FASD training the following year would spotlight the need for FASD to be included in SSI. His savings could supplement him for now until SSI was available, God willing.

I left for the trip, feeling relieved to have finally gotten away, but also a bit apprehensive about leaving Nicky. While I was gone, I tried to call him several times, but he didn't respond. I checked in with my mother, and she hadn't seen him either, although they were supposed to have dinner together. This wasn't like Nicky, as he was always dependable. Something was off.

When I came home a few days later, I walked into a quiet house. There was a note on my desk.

Nicky had left home.

Saying that things weren't going well and work wasn't what he thought it should be, he had gone to live elsewhere and would call me when he got settled in.

Reading these words knocked the breath out of me. Wondering where he had gone and who had influenced him to leave, I began wracking my brain about where he could be and how this could have happened. Although I knew something was up and I needed to talk with him, I didn't expect this. At the same time, how in the heck could he have just left, sneaky as all get-out?

I ran up to his room. His suitcase and clothes were missing, but the majority of his treasured belongings were still in his room, as well as a laundry basket full of dirty clothes.

How could he leave without his beloved bowling balls? And he left his dirty laundry? How dare he! I was scared and furious and distraught and pissed off that I had another mess to clean up and figure out!

As angry as I was, I was frightened and knew he could end up in a bad situation he didn't see coming. There's nothing that can prepare a parent when an adult child runs away from home. The parent's hands are tied as well because that child is a legal adult and allowed to make his own decisions!

Immediately, I got in my car and headed to the grocery store down the street where he worked, calling his best friend, Scott, at the same time. Scott and Nicky's friendship was solid. Scott was very loyal to Nicky and was a wonderful influence of friendship and faith.

"Scott, this is Ms. Jacobus. I just got home and Nicky is gone. Do you know where he is?"

"Yes, well, no, sort of, I mean both. I know he's gone. I

think he went to live with his brother. He wasn't happy at work, and he felt he needed to live on his own but he couldn't. Also, there's a guy at work who just moved into his own place and that might have influenced Nicky. I've been telling Nicky for months to talk to you."

In shock and trying to collect my thoughts, I couldn't speak. Scott continued talking.

"I didn't think he was actually serious about leaving. We were supposed to go out the night he left. I didn't know he was gone until I called him, and he was already at the airport."

"Scott, did you say you think he went to live with his brother?"

"Yes, that's right."

Good God, they were just here. Why didn't they say anything to me? Nicky could have gone out there for a long visit and cleared it with work. I would have been fine with that. In fact, I needed the break, too!

"Scott, I just got to his work. I'm going to talk to them, and I'll call you back."

I called my oldest son before going into the store, but there was no answer. I left a voice message.

At the customer service desk, I asked if Nicky had worked over the weekend. They told me that he hadn't shown up for work for a few days and didn't call in. It would be noted as "abandonment." In other words, he was fired and would have no medical insurance, no job references, and no income. I talked with the store manager, who said Nicky was very likable and was helpful to the customers, though he was easily distracted and had to be brought back on task. Still, the store manager said he was like family, and they would do whatever was possible to help. They were so sorry to see him gone and asked me to keep them informed if I heard from the "prodigal son."

How in the heck could he have just left without giving them a two-week notice? At least he could have been respectful to the people he'd worked with for eight years. He was leaving work benefits he had earned, his customers, and friends. Obviously, not much thinking had gone into the great escape.

If he was living with his brother, how in the heck could they have agreed to this? How could anyone have steered him in that direction? If he wanted to try living with his brother, he could have taken a leave of absence. No problem! Just don't leave without employment and insurance. That's foolish! Here I was, swirling in dysfunctional chaos that had swallowed our family again!

I called my son. No answer. Called Nicky's phone, no answer.

I was pacing the floor trying to figure out where he was and what had happened when the phone rang. It was Nicky's brother.

"Hi, Mom."

"Where is Nicky?"

"He's with me."

"How did he get out there?"

"He got a ticket and flew out here. He was on the phone with me the whole time so he didn't get lost. He did it and is fine."

"Fine, he's fine. Well, it isn't fine! He left his job without any notice. It's called 'abandonment.'"

"I told him to call his work when he got here."

"I'd say that was a little too late since they'd have to find someone to replace him. Now he has no benefits, insurance, or references. Eight years of employment and his 'shining star' employee recognition is now moot as he's been fired!

"He'll be my dependent."

"Your dependent . . . really? He's twenty-six years old. And he has a disability. I've been trying to get him SSI, which he doesn't qualify for. In the meantime, he needed to be employed with full medical benefits. He's not your dependent and is over the age of dependency. As an adult he needs his diagnosis re-evaluated, along with the lengthy process of lots of paperwork. It should have been done before he went out there. He's left family, friends, and coworkers without even saying goodbye."

"Well, I need you to send his ID papers, Social Security card, passport, and all of his diagnosis papers."

Trying to keep my anger in check, I said, "I am about to say some things that I wouldn't normally say and hope I never have to say again. *What in the hell were you thinking?* I have worked my ass off for twenty years to take care of him, keep him insured, get him on a path of progression, and do what's necessary to help him with his disability. I'm not going to have you pluck him from home and ask for all of the things that I worked so damn hard to get. He's got his important file folder with copies of his ID information, which will be accessible to get anything he needs. You have to apply for your own originals. I'm not releasing any of the originals to have them lost and have to redo it all when he returns. If you think you can take care of him, then prove it by applying for those papers. Just like I did."

"Mom, to get him as a dependent I'm going to need you to send the papers."

"No, you don't! What happens when people lose their papers or they're stolen? I've gone through both with you kids. I had to reapply for them. You can do the same thing."

He was silent, and I was trying to catch my breath. The fire of anger that was raging seemed to be snuffing out the oxygen I needed to breathe, and I was in disbelief at what I was hearing from him.

"I can't even talk to you anymore. Call me when you make sense." I hung up the phone.

I was fuming.

It was understandable why Nicky was not happy at home or in his job. He'd had twenty years of cabin fever, I get it. But this was not the way to do it. I felt so sucker-punched and betrayed by both of them.

Just as I'd navigated life for Nicky, I'd done the same thing for his older brother. I never gave in or gave up on him. For him not to trust me enough to contact me about the huge mistake they were making was incomprehensible.

In addition to Nicky no longer having a job or health insurance or even the camaraderie of his beloved bowling team, I feared he would be exposed to alcohol and might fall into behaviors he had, so far, avoided. It was unlikely he'd have the protective factors he needed to safely navigate life's choices while living elsewhere.

While Nicky was spending time with his brother during the summer homecoming visit, Nicky had mentioned his brother's drinking. Concerned, but knowing Nicky's dislike for the behaviors he's seen resulting from alcohol, I encouraged him to stand firm, don't drink, and also never get into a vehicle with someone who's been drinking.

During the next few months, there was little contact with Nicky or his brother. I prayed Nicky was safe and doing well and not participating in behaviors that would be harmful to him. As time went on, I continued to call Nicky many times only to have the conversations cut short. I tried to get him home to collect his things, but he said he had to stay at his brother's home. They would be vacationing out of the country and needed him to care for their pets. Not a good idea. If something happened while they were gone, what was Nicky to do? Call his brother for help and they would walk across the street from whatever country they were in to help him?

On one occasion I spoke with Nicky, he revealed that he and his brother had gotten drunk several times. Now I was concerned Nicky would participate in high risk behaviors, such as tattooing, vaping, and smoking. With his impairment in judgment, these behaviors would jeopardize his finances and his ability to recognize the three basic needs of food, clothing, and shelter. After a short, gentle lecture from me about the dangers of alcohol, he rarely took my calls. Shortly thereafter, his phone, that I was paying for, was sent back to me. No note, no explanation. There was no way to contact him to find out what was going on.

And then there was the money. He had access to his checking/savings account with plenty of money at his disposal, but his additional savings account was in a secure account being managed by my financial adviser and making a good amount of interest, all for his future. There was no way anyone was getting their hands on it until I could put it securely in Nicky's hands.

I began receiving emails from his brother saying Nicky would only talk to me if I sent him his savings account. Had they not yet experienced any of Nicky's challenges to understand that his money was being kept safe for him? He'd get it when he came home and made arrangements to leave responsibly. How could they think I was going to agree to this nonsense? Yeah, that would happen when hell freezes over *or* he came home to retrieve the rest of his belongings, including his dirty laundry.

I guess hell was about to freeze.

Chapter 30

Failure to Launch

It was a new year and the freezing cold weather had set in.

There was still no word from Nicky, and my concern was that even the CliffsNotes version of his invisible disability wasn't being addressed by his new caregivers.

That's the problem. People who aren't caregivers don't know how exhausting it can be to create a normal life for those with an FASD—and they don't know how mind-boggling it is to maintain that normal life. It all seems normal to outsiders looking in.

It bears repeating. Navigating life for those with an FASD has challenges beyond what people on the outside can even perceive.

Yet, with the right environmental prescription and life coaching, those with FASD can lead happy, productive lives. Yes, it's hard, but there's hope.

Five months had passed, and Nicky was probably frustrated living with a baby and not getting his needs met by a brother who was busy with his wife, work, and child. It can take a toll on a family, putting relationships in turmoil because different personalities have different ways of addressing challenges. The idea is not to work harder but work smarter, and in unison. Many people don't have time for this.

In the last conversation I had with Nicky, he mentioned his brother and his family would be on vacation in the winter months, leaving Nicky behind to take care of the home front for a few weeks. It was not a good idea, and there was nothing I could do about it. Natural consequences would take their course, sooner or later.

Well, it was sooner.

It was the end of January, and I received an email from my oldest son saying Nicky needed to find another home. Apparently, Nicky was behaving in ways that could be interpreted as threatening to their baby. Knowing Nicky's impulsive remarks could be misinterpreted, I suspected he didn't want a baby monopolizing his brother's time. I'd seen this myself on occasion with his sister's baby. Nicky didn't want to be pestered by the baby's crying or typical baby needs. It was a harmless reaction, but perhaps not to a new mother whose job was to protect and nurture her infant. And caring for an infant and caring for a person with challenges takes a whole lot of patience—a lot to place on a new mother, who might not be prepared. Understandably, living with his brother and his family wasn't going to work with Nicky acting out in this way.

I tried to call them but only managed to get through with email. I offered to help and tried to rest their fears about Nicky's behavior. There was no response.

Weeks and months went by without correspondence. I was busy traveling for FASD presentations, and the time passed quickly. Nicky's birthday was at the end of March; in the past, we'd spent it going to the airport, having lunch, and watching the planes. We'd done it for years. It was a favorite day for Nicky, and I enjoyed giving him this as a birthday gift. The sky was the limit on this day. Nicky loved planes and was fascinated with space.

This year, I was only able to send him a birthday card, which I prayed he would receive. I didn't know if he was even still living with his brother. I sent the birthday card certified, signature required, return receipt, by Nicky only. The return receipt came back with a signature, though it was not Nicky's. Shortly thereafter I received an email saying that Nicky was fine. But again, it included a demand to send the money from his savings account before I could have any contact with him. I responded to the request, again, that this would only happen when Nicky returned home to retrieve his belongings and to say his proper goodbyes. If things were working out with their living arrangements, great! I just needed him safe and happy. The money would be available upon his returning for a visit home. I never got an answer.

I went out of town for another work trip, and when I returned home a week later, I learned Nicky was back in Georgia. The tip was from an unlikely source, but one who cared about Nicky. *Where was he? How long had he been back? Was he safe, happy, and why the heck had he not called me?*

It's not so easy to try to guide someone into independent living when they need supportive housing and an external brain to help them. Interdependent living. It sure looks easy on the outside, but just have a little taste of what it's really like to try to teach someone who's resistant to the help that's needed. It can quickly become unmanageable, especially when the caregiver doesn't have the right environmental prescription.

In this case, Nicky had failed to launch.

However, at this point I wasn't worried about a failed launch but a train wreck ready to happen!

Chapter 31

The Train Wreck

Nicky's train had apparently pulled into his dad's station. Nicky was safe, living with his dad, and working at his company. I was relieved.

My communication with his dad was limited. In earlier conversations with DS, he had told me I was the source of Nicky's challenges because I was too overprotective and kept his boundaries too restricted. For my part, I was fearful Nicky would be at risk because DS didn't understand the protective factors Nicky needed to be safe and stable.

Just like Nicky needed a prescription for glasses to help him see clearly, he needed an environmental prescription to help him navigate life. Tragically, some people think if they don't need help navigating through life, no one else does either. That's like saying just because one person doesn't need glasses, no one else needs them. Nicky needed routine, schedule, and structure to help him make decisions and see how to properly navigate life.

Again, FASD is an invisible disability and not everyone can see it.

When I called his dad's company to talk with Nicky, one of the staff members put me through.

"Hello."

"Hi Nicky, it's Mom. How are you?"

"I'm fine."

"It's great you're working at the company! I've been concerned about you. I wish you would have called me to let me know you were okay. How long have you been back?"

"I'm fine, Mom. Been here awhile."

"Are you living with Pop?"

"Yep."

"Good, and you like your job?"

"Yep."

It was evident from his responses he wasn't interested in talking to me. Needing to make my point quickly that the door was always open for him to come home, it was obvious it wasn't going to happen anytime soon. Still, I was relieved he was safe, under his dad's roof, and employed.

"Mom, I want my money, will you send it to me?"

"Not a problem. Just come by the house to get your things and we'll go to the bank to transfer it to you."

"Can't you just send it in a check?"

"No, I'm not going to mail it. It could get lost. Come by and we'll go to the bank, and all of it will be transferred to you. Next week would be a good time. Looking forward to seeing you and I'm glad you're safe. Love you."

"Okay, Mom. Bye."

And that was it. Distant and detached after almost twenty years of nurturing, guiding, and enduring after adopting him at age five. But I knew I'd have to step in again somewhere along the line to clean up the inevitable.

Hell thawed on a warm June day when, after some convincing, Nicky came by to pick up his belongings, and we visited the bank to transfer his money. He brought a friend I hadn't met. He was kind, helping Nicky pack up, and saw that Nicky had not grown up attached to a ball and chain. I didn't have to convince him of this fact, he could see it on the family pictures hanging on the walls, and how Nicky was now reminiscing about his childhood, sharing fond memories. I glanced at his friend, and he seemed to understand I was hoping he knew I wasn't the beast Nicky might have portrayed me to be. I thanked him for his help, and he reached out with a reassuring hug. I then hugged Nicky but kept my words to a minimum, just letting him know I loved him.

I didn't know when I would talk to or see him again. He was on his own, but I'd begin preparing a safety net.

The calls from Nicky were few. I would call him, leaving messages about once a week, offering lunch or dinner to let him know I cared. I was grateful he was not living on the street, but living with his dad. Perhaps his father would see for himself that Nicky needed help, and perhaps he would assist him. Though hurt I wasn't his go-to person when Nicky arrived back in Georgia, I was relieved to know he was safe, living with his dad, employed, and had medical benefits.

This put my mind at ease, and I redirected my energy to the upcoming FASD training in September, as the work was mounting. The FASD experts would be staying at my home, and I turned my basement into an FASD processing plant of paperwork, promotional items, and folders to stuff. A couple of friends, Teresa and Becky, who understood the needs of my kids, knew I was stretched beyond my capabilities with pulling this thing off and jumped in at the final hour. Thank God. To prepare for the event, my mother would help assemble training packets and bake homemade breakfast items, and Natalia would be making southern peach cobbler. It was all coming together.

The State Bar of Georgia was the venue. Dedicated sponsors, such as the Georgia Office of the Child Advocate, were on board, lending their support to address this much-needed cause. The timing was perfect. Natalia had completed her probation's community service and payment of fines and restitution and would also be present, distributing the information training bags to attendees. Dedicated friends had offered their help and time. I prayed Nicky would be at the training—he knew the importance of it firsthand. Perhaps Maurice would be there also. I had continued searching for him throughout that year and found nothing. Was he living on the street, lost, or supported by caregivers? Praying for the latter, I was just thankful Nicky was safe, as he could have been in a situation similar to Maurice's, the unknown.

The FASD training was well-received. FASD experts

Billy Edwards, Dr. Larry Burd, Dr. Paul Conner, Dr. Doug Waite, and Tom Donaldson brought their top-notch expertise to Atlanta. The presenters' personal stories were touching, relatable, and highly informative, as was their commitment to make a difference. The local resources and sponsors did the same. God was again providing a shoulder to lean on in the form of incredible people coming together to advocate for those unable to help themselves. Natalia was a gem. I was so proud of her and her willingness to share her story. The attendees spoke to her during the event to learn about the challenges and successes she'd experienced. The attendees also learned about how her FASD secondary conditions, which contributed to her challenges of impulsivity and vulnerability, had landed her in trouble with the law three years earlier. We couldn't have imagined that only a week after the FASD training, she would need assistance from some of those very same people, who now had a better understanding of her disability. She was navigating, progressing, and acknowledging her disability and shortcomings. She was working through it all with humility and taking ownership of her decisions and disability. She is a gift and an inspiration.

Throughout the summer, little bits and pieces of Nicky's challenging behaviors were emerging. He told me he had purchased a car in June and had already totaled it after losing control on a winding road and hitting a tree. Thank God he wasn't injured, nor was anyone else. He said he had no car insurance, which wasn't noted on the police report. He had the insurance card but said the insurance company didn't "take" his first payment. That made no sense and a whole lot of other things were beginning to make no sense as he and I met a few times to check in. This included the money I had transferred to him. It was nearly gone, and there were no "checks and balances" on where it had gone. Nicky didn't keep track of the money in a checkbook register like he'd been taught growing up. Now it was all virtual and digital, which for him was out of sight, out of mind.

As for his transportation, he was already driving another car, which wasn't being maintained properly. He told me he would soon be living with someone he met on Craigslist, instead of his dad.

This was a red flag! Who would be overseeing his daily life navigational system? Who would provide his protective factors? Who would furnish his environmental prescription?

My gut instinct that trouble was ramping up was strong. Something seemed off. We were in touch for a week, then a few more weeks went by with no contact. Then one day I called and got a recording saying his phone was no longer in working order. He had either lost his phone, it had been stolen, or he had not paid his bill.

Well, it was reassuring that at least he was still working for his dad's company.

When I tried to call Nicky at work, I was told he had not been there for about three weeks. It was evident he had lost his job. I said I was Nicky's mother and asked for Nicky's home address. The woman I was speaking with said she didn't have one on record. She didn't seem to understand the seriousness of the situation and was short with her answers as I pleaded for her to help me. She was acting as if she was shielding him from an overprotective mother. She even said Nicky didn't seem to have a disability. I told her I'd lived with my son for twenty years and understood full well his disability, whether she thought he had one or not. The line went dead.

Yet another person had been fooled by this invisible disability.

Immediately calling her back, I asked if the call had dropped, and she admitted she hung up on me. Although frustrated, I knew this was not the time for me to be confrontational. I needed information about Nicky, and I was going to uncover every stone, even if the stone was jagged! I apologized if I had offended her and told her I was worried about Nicky and to please call me if she was able to find the address where he was living or if he called in. She accepted my apology and we hung up. It was a dead end.

I reached out to his dad that afternoon, emailing him with questions about what had happened to Nicky and where he was living. I pictured Nicky in some rundown apartment and not capable of getting himself out of his own mess, but thinking he could. This was the pattern of his behavior, evident even when he was a little boy, and he needed consistent guidance to make good choices.

Supportive people who understand his needs are his compass. If he doesn't have that, he could go down the wrong path, into homelessness or criminal behavior to survive.

There was no response from his dad. It was a dead end, again.

I called Nicky's good friend Scott. He also hadn't heard from Nicky and had been trying to contact him. I called several other of Nicky's friends. No one had heard from him. They were all on board, sharing their concern, and offering to help me in any way possible. Thank God he had these friends who cared about him and understood the seriousness of the situation.

After a sleepless Friday night, and still no response from Nicky's dad, I called him early the next morning, threatening to show up on his doorstep unless I got answers. DS said Nicky had possibly driven to Texas to meet up with a friend he'd made while living with his brother. The confusing story continued. There was something about Nicky not being able to pay rent to his new landlord, but he was coming into a large sum of money via the internet and would pay it as soon as he could.

That would be an internet scam!

Nicky was in trouble. Without his environmental prescription, he was at risk. He was driving a car that needed maintenance, had unlimited use of a smart phone, which can expose him to the toxic underworld, and he'd fallen prey to both. Stranded by one and risking incarceration from the other if he wasn't found soon. He needed help!

And why hadn't I been told he was missing?!

Nicky had had lots of time to make his own choices while living with his brother and his father. It didn't work. They don't see his challenges and don't think he needs support, a.k.a. "glasses." In the meantime, Nicky was out on the street somewhere!

Here it was October 13, and Nicky had possibly been on the street for three weeks. Had I known, I would have already been in my car three weeks ago looking for him. Well, we know what can happen in three weeks. I'd already gone through it with Natalia. This was not going to happen with Nicky, too.

I called and left messages for my oldest son. He provided limited information, was distant and detached. I was furious that they were aware Nicky was missing and had not contacted me. Nicky was at risk. It was gut-wrenching. I moved on to other resources, which would prove to be more helpful. We all needed to work together to find him.

God knows what Nicky had said about me when he first went to live with his brother or his dad. That he lived in a bubble and had no freedom to make his own choices? Yeah, it was a real hellhole! When he got the freedom they thought he should have, look where it led. Freedom is available when Nicky takes healthy ownership of his choices and has a responsible understanding of consequences. When he has challenges without understanding the consequences, coupled with poor judgment, he ends up in harm's way! He needs help navigating life with safe boundaries and protective factors.

233

Read his file!

Frustrated beyond belief, I wanted to crawl into a dark hole, which right about then was more desirable than the work needed to find him. Exhaustion was setting in. Praying that God would somehow replace the helplessness I was feeling with a glimmer of light, direction, and hope, I remembered the help I'd received in the past from a private investigator friend of mine. She was sharp, resourceful, and undeniably candid.

My brain was an emotional mess and clarity was needed. When I called her, she pointed me in the right direction, and the light went on! With her no-nonsense approach, she told me to take the *##% emotion out of the moment and prioritize the task! She probably would have slapped me on the side of the head, saying, "Snap out of it!" if she had been standing next to me. Jolted by her strong, authoritative voice and specific step-by-step instructions, I needed to pull it together and file a missing persons report as soon as possible.

To file the report, the police would need the address of the last place Nicky was living—first with his father, then in an apartment with someone he had found on the internet. They would also need the tag number on his car to track his vehicle.

I emailed Nicky's dad, requesting the information. He shot back a response saying he didn't have it, and Nicky hadn't provided it to the company.

Funny thing, previously, Nicky had told me his dad had

helped him find his apartment and had even met with the landlord. I emailed DS again that evening and called him the following morning, promising I'd camp out on his doorstep until I got some answers. Finally, he emailed me the address where Nicky had been living. He also told me he was on his way there to pick up Nicky's belongings, which would be placed on the curb because Nicky was being evicted.

Dashing out the door, I planned to meet with the landlord, but more importantly, pick up Nicky's things to search for clues to his whereabouts, as it would be a starting point to find him.

I was too late.

DS called to say he had already picked up Nicky's possessions, and I would have to meet him at his office to retrieve anything. This was not what I wanted to hear.

I rerouted to the office. He was waiting for me in the parking lot with a truck full of Nicky's belongings. I asked to take all the belongings with me. He didn't agree, so I had to rummage through to get what I needed. I was informed any documents I took had to be photocopied. I then headed to the landlord's (a.k.a. the evictor's) house where Nicky had lived for a short time.

The "evictor's" real name was similar to the iconic singer Marvin Gaye, and I couldn't help but think how ironic it was that I was wondering what was going on and could definitely use some mercy. When I drove up to his house and pulled into his driveway, the evictor was on guard, walking up toward me with another man.

"Can I help you?"

"Hi, yes. I'm looking for Nicky."

"Who?"

"Nicky. I'm his mother."

"I don't know a Nicky."

Confused that perhaps I was at the wrong address, I remembered that after Nicky left home, he'd decided he wanted to be known by his formal name, as he was embarrassed by his nickname, "Nicky." It wasn't a common name, and to Nicky, it sounded like a girl's name, and he'd been teased about it.

"I'm sorry, that's his nickname. His given name is Nicholas."

"Yes, I'm familiar with him."

I would soon find out the landlord's cautious demeanor hid his kindness. I gave him my contact card in case he heard anything from Nicky. I apologized for the abrupt visit and the confusion. He apologized for the unwelcoming attitude. He said an hour earlier, he had been warned by his previous visitor, Nicky's dad, that I might be coming by to "interrogate" him.

Interrogate him? The puzzle pieces of Nicky's whereabouts needed to be put together. This wasn't the time to be a milquetoast. After twenty years of advocating on behalf of my kids, I learned to put that milk carton away. Nicky's face was not about to appear on one, either!

The landlord looked at my card, and asked about Nicky's mental state, telling me he and the tenants in the house had detected a possible disability, though they couldn't pinpoint it. I explained Nicky's challenges with FASD, and the landlord nodded thankfully in understanding. He got it! He said if he had known about Nicky's FASD challenges, he and his roommates could have looked out for him.

The man who was with the landlord overheard our discussion and politely interrupted to ask about FASD. He then asked me for any information I could provide, as his son was arriving in the next couple of weeks from out of state. His son was in his early twenties, adopted, and had multiple challenges. He indicated his son was on the FASD spectrum. It was amazing that in all the chaos of trying to find Nicky, this man needed to learn more about FASD to help his son when he arrived. And some people are in denial that FASD exists? It's a pandemic!

I gave him FASD literature while I tried to absorb all the information the landlord had shared about his three weeks with Nicky. They had a good relationship and liked him. It was a relief to know Nicky had been in good hands. The landlord offered to help in any way he could. He gave me an updated picture of Nicky and even offered to go with me to the police station to file the missing persons report.

Thanking him, and being thankful for him, I left knowing he and I would be in contact if we heard anything from Nicky.

Making the hour-long drive back home, I prayed Nicky was safe. Tomorrow was going to be busy. The suspected train wreck was a reality, and the scattered pieces to find him seemed to be strewn all over the place.

Nicky was officially missing, and the gut-wrenching feeling I had, wondering how he would be found, was beyond what I was prepared for.

Chapter 32

BOLO

The next morning the gut-wrenching feeling was still there. Nicky was missing somewhere between Texas and Georgia, possibly near Tuscaloosa, Alabama. At this point the situation seemed worse than looking for a needle in a haystack. The leads were minimal, if not nonexistent. My prayers would continue, and many friends were on board, offering to help find him.

Looking at this overwhelming haystack, my first step was to find his car tag. The police department needed it for the missing persons report I would file later that day, and the police report had to be filed in the county where he was last living, so I would be heading right back to where I was the day before. My friend, the private investigator, explained I also had to check Nicky's phone and bank records, which would include ATM locations. As I'd learned a few years earlier when searching for Natalia, this was exhausting. These companies don't put enough security measures in place to prevent criminal activity and protect their customers, then make it extremely difficult to access information to help customers after they've become victims. It's another wild goose chase. I could either sit around twiddling my thumbs or try to find the information.

Sitting around doing nothing was not an option. I'd already found car repair invoices and bank account information the day before when I'd searched through Nicky's possessions that were in his dad's truck.

The dilemma was not knowing if he even had a current car tag. A similar situation had occurred when Nicky thought he had car insurance, but he had never followed through to make the first payment. Did he even have a car tag and did he actually put it on his car? If his dad had told him what to do, thinking he would follow through, he might not have done it. Although I expected my kids to follow through on simple requests, they wouldn't necessarily do them, especially if they were distracted.

I remember our family social worker telling me to watch our children do the task or complete it with them. The more the children experienced completing the task, with repetition, those behaviors became habits.

I returned to the papers I'd found, looking for anything that might give me his car tag. I was interrupted by a call from one of my closest friends. Hearing her voice, I broke down in tears. Teresa knew the challenges of the past twenty years, and she was always available to lend an ear and sound advice. We wracked our brains, hers not mine, as mine was depleted, as we dissected Nicky's last car repair invoice. Good Lord, so much work was recommended. The car should never have been driven out of state! I took the information on the repair invoice and registered it on a website that provides a service report history for vehicles. The last repairs were from the invoice I had in hand. Most importantly, the VIN number was also there, so I could call the county where the car was registered to possibly find the tag number.

Not knowing which county the car was registered in, I had to call the tag offices in the several counties where Nicky had lived. Three times was the charm, and I was finally speaking to the tax commissioner in one of these counties, explaining to her that my son was missing and his car was broken down somewhere between Texas and Georgia. She must have heard the despair in my voice, and because I had provided her with enough information to look up the records, she found and shared the tag number. She was another angel that was needed to find Nicky.

With the tag number in hand, I headed to the police department an hour away to file the missing persons report. On the way, I stopped by the landlord's home because he had offered to provide a recent photo of Nicky and give me a few more of Nicky's belongings that were accidently left behind. He also shared some information he'd received from DS the day before, indicating that I was responsible for Nicky's challenges and my advocacy efforts were self-promotion.

Although I was shocked, the many psych evaluations completed on my kids spoke for themselves. When someone has a disability, they need the proper tools to help them. Bringing FASD awareness to educators and counselors and providing the environmental prescription of a safe, structured, living space *is* providing these tools. Teaching Nicky to advocate for himself and understand his own strengths and weaknesses prepares him for his future. It was evident, again, this disability is so invisible that many can't see it.

This further demonstrated his father's denial and lack of understanding about FASD—another reason why it needs to be officially documented and recognized in the medical community. If the parent of a child with FASD doesn't recognize it, how can society recognize it and support them? We needed more FASD education and awareness, with an increased screening for prenatal alcohol exposure and improved diagnosis of FASD. Every state should recognize FASD as a developmental disability.

Ironically, when I'd met DS at his office the day before to search through some of Nicky's belongings, he told me he had tried to teach Nicky how to budget, and Nicky couldn't grasp any of it. Frustrated, he said he explained it to him repeatedly, and he still didn't get it! He said Nicky had also misused his phone by accessing paid content and was obstinate when his father corrected him about these behaviors. He said Nicky was a know-it-all and wouldn't listen.

He asked me, "How can he not get it?"

"Maybe the same way you don't get it?"

It's exhausting to bring these behaviors to the forefront while you're butting heads with those who are in denial and saying nothing is wrong—it's just willful behavior. Okay, when someone has a peanut allergy, should we just expect them to eat peanuts because others can? You can't see the peanut allergy! But if someone who is allergic to peanuts eats them, it can be life-threatening.

Educating society about a little-to-unknown disorder so kids don't end up homeless or in jail is advocacy. Advocating on their behalf is their lifeline.

Thank God the landlord got it and was supportive, willing to help Nicky with whatever he could.

Another of God's angels, helping me find Nicky.

As I drove to the police department I was relieved, thinking the missing persons report would be fairly easy to file in comparison to finding out where Nicky had lived. His name, a photo, recent address, car make and model, and tag number. What else could they possibly need except a few of his friends' phone numbers, which I also had. Feeling prepared and ready to provide all that was needed, I was good to go!

Apparently, I spoke too soon. To file the missing persons report, I should have known what Nicky was wearing the last time I saw him, which was about a month ago. Stupid me, how could I not remember what he was wearing a month ago. Imagine that! Boy, oh boy, apparently what he was wearing a month ago was a sure-fire way to find him, and I needed every detail about his shirt color and style of pants to complete the report to find him. God help us all if he had changed his clothes. Even the recent photo, car make and model, and information about his disability weren't as important! It seemed the details of what he was wearing were the key to finding Nicky.

The officer writing up the report was not what I expected as he still seemed to be wet behind the ears. While I explained Nicky had an invisible disability, the officer ignored what I said and explained he couldn't put out a BOLO ("be on the lookout") because he couldn't see his disability in the photo. Did I not just say he had an "invisible disability"? Even though I showed him documentation of Nicky's disability and how it related to Nicky's behavior and his inability to keep himself out of harm's way, he still couldn't grasp how important it was to find him. Frustrated and knowing I wasn't going to waste any more time providing this officer with information he couldn't understand, I made up a description of what clothes Nicky might have been wearing, and I kept my answers short, which was very difficult for me to do. The report was filed. It would be a few days before I could access the police report, and a detective wouldn't be calling me for a week or so.

I left knowing I wasn't going to wait for the police. I would be in my car early the next morning and on my way to Tuscaloosa, Alabama, to do my own detective work.

That night, yet again, I got on those trusted knees in prayer.

By the grace of God, Nicky would be found and it wouldn't be too late.

Chapter 33

By the Grace of God

Four years earlier, I'd driven an hour to a drug-ridden hotel to find clues to Natalia's whereabouts. This time it would be a six-hour, faith-driven ride to find Nicky.

I was tired, not in the best condition to be driving on the highway while looking for a broken-down car or an unrecognizable kid walking the streets, possibly holding one of those "Will work for food" signs. Praying before I left my house, I asked God to make this a heck of a lot easier than what I went through to find Natalia.

My prayers were passionate and pleading.

"God, please give me easy—"

My phone rang.

Thank God, He was listening. It was my friend Evan, who would not let me go at this alone. He eventually convinced me to let him drive, so I could keep my eyes peeled to the side of the road for six hours, looking for Nicky.

We left the house before the sun came up to avoid Atlanta's rush hour traffic.

The longer car ride might allow me more time to strategize how to find him, though it would also allow me more time to ruminate with worry about what the circumstances might be. And *if* he is found, *will* he come home?

Unlike the situation with Natalia, Diane wasn't there, and it was unlikely a SWAT team would show up to help. I would, however, call the Tuscaloosa police department to give them a heads-up, as Nicky could be hanging out on a park bench, in whatever clothes he was wearing, which were undoubtedly not the same clothes from a month earlier.

Shuffling through Nicky's belongings I'd brought with me, I found an inconspicuous piece of paper listing hotel phone numbers in Texas. I began calling these hotels where Nicky might have been. All these options needed to be excluded as this faith-driven ride continued.

I was interrupted by a call from a couple of concerned friends. They would be praying for his safe return also.

All hotels on the list for Texas were called. No Nicky!

As my friend was driving the family car, the dependable, trusted Yukon with over two hundred thousand miles on it, I scanned the side of the road. This old family car had taken good care of us on vacations, school events, and trips to the emergency room for broken bones. On more than one occasion we had used it to transport more than sixteen bales of pine straw for our wonderful, relaxing weekends of yard work. This car had seen plenty of long-distance trips, caring for us through the years, and was like a member of the family that could be easily recognized. Nicky had a special bond with this car, as he was the one who most often washed it and cleaned the tires well. There was something very quirky about Nicky's relationship with car tires! I was thankful the car was still in good working order and recognizable.

Needing to stop for gas, the timing was perfect as we were crossing into Tuscaloosa.

The gas station was attached to what looked to be a local convenience store and hangout. It was a little sketchy, but there was a police car in the parking lot. We decided to go in for coffee and food, and there was an officer waiting for the next available cashier. Evan encouraged me to inundate the officer with my own BOLO report. I scurried after the officer as he walked to his patrol car. Good Lord, this certainly beats having to find the Tuscaloosa police department when my time would be better spent searching the streets for Nicky. God was making this easier!

As I filled the officer in on what had transpired in the last three weeks, including a description and photo of Nicky, the officer wrote down the information in detail, asking a few questions. He was not familiar with anyone living on the street who matched that description, but he assured me he would immediately share the information with others to help find Nicky.

As Evan and I drove through Tuscaloosa to the outskirts of the city, our starting point was to go to every hotel, garage, and auto repair shop. To bolster my credibility, I'd brought along photos of Nicky and articles about our FASD advocacy efforts. One of the photos was Nicky with the governor of Georgia. Now that's credibility!

Driving to the outskirts of the city, passing many repair shops, we made a U-turn to come back into the city where several roads crossed over each other, making it difficult to know which one Nicky might have taken, if he had even traveled on it.

The pull to take one road over another was strong, with no real reason. A repair shop was off in the distance but a hotel was straight ahead. Driving into the hotel parking lot, neither Nicky nor his car was there. Heading back to the highway onto another road, there were many repair shops. But the repair shop that had caught my attention was off in the distance and not easy to get to. Again, a pull to go to this repair shop was evident to me, and I insisted that we make a beeline and cut through a few parking lots to get there. It looked like a used-car lot or perhaps a repair shop with many old, beat-up cars. Nevertheless, it would be our first stop among a whole slew we would make to find Nicky. Jumping out of the car, armed with photos, articles, and the police report, and leaving my friend behind with the motor running, I entered the repair shop. The smell of engine oil and cigarettes filled the room.

"Hi, ma'am. May I help you with something?"

"Yes, I'm looking for my son. His car broke down somewhere between Texas and here, and no one has heard from him in weeks. I've filed a missing person's report in Atlanta. Here is a recent picture of him."

Taking a deep breath, I handed him the picture.

"Have you seen him?"

At this point a few of the workers had walked into the shop to check out what was happening. Looking at their bewildered faces, I couldn't tell if I would be escorted out of the shop or if they were in disbelief.

That's when I realized what it was: there was a palpable feeling in the room of being witness to something miraculous.

The man looked at me, looked down at the picture, and up at me again.

"Well, ma'am, yes, this is Nicholas."

He didn't say this looks like Nicholas, this could be Nicholas, or I recognize this boy.

He knew Nicky!

"His car is broken down. It's sitting on the back lot behind this building, and he's living out there on the street."

He was confident, no question about it!

Overwhelmed and holding back tears of relief, I began questioning him.

"He's here? Where? When is the last time you saw him?"

"He was just here this morning, checking out that Mustang for sale over there. He thinks he's going to be able to buy it once he gets enough money saved up, then head back to where he came from. Ma'am, he sure is a nice boy, polite and all, but something just doesn't seem right with the way he's thinking. And his car, he never should have been driving it. It's a run-down mess. Engine's blown. Car isn't worth hardly anything, and he owes me money for towing it off the street."

"Can I see the car to make sure it's his? I need to find him—where did you say he was living?"

"He was living on the street, but I think for the last couple of nights he's been staying over there at the Salvation Army."

"Can I take one of your business cards? And here's mine. I'll be back to take care of the expenses for his car, but I need to find him first."

Running out to the car where I had left my friend, he rolled down the window.

"Nicky's here. Well, not here, but they have his car. Come with me to make sure it's his."

Evan stared at me, ignoring what I was saying. He thought I was teasing. As he waited for me to get in the car, he took the gear out of park to quickly go onto the next stop.

"No, really, he's here. His car is out back, and I need you to come check it out."

"He's what? Here? How can that be possible?"

"His car is here, come on. We need to find him. He might be at the Salvation Army."

Checking the back lot, we found Nicky's car. The car tag was on it and his belongings were inside. I went back inside the repair shop and assured the owner that we'd be back once we found him. He said he was not concerned about the car expenses and told us to go find Nicky. If Nicky stopped by the garage, they had my phone number and would immediately call me.

After a short drive down the road, we pulled into the Salvation Army. Leaving my friend to wait in the car, I took only the most recent picture of Nicky. The attendant at the front desk greeted me, and she looked at the picture but couldn't give me any information if he had been staying at their facility, company policy. I'd been down that road before with the privacy laws that seem to work against parents trying to find their adult children.

I needed to use the mom card. If that didn't work, I would use the governor card! Running back to the car to get the articles written about Nicky being spotlighted by the Centers for Disease Control (CDC) for his ability to overcome his FASD challenges, along with several other articles about our family's advocacy, I shared them with her. I believe it was the photo of the governor and Nicky that caught her eye. Ok, maybe it was a mom's desperation! After seeing all the photos, the woman behind the desk got up from her seat and walked to the front door, telling me to follow her. Outside, she put her arm around my shoulder and pointed at a park.

"Please listen to me very carefully. I can't tell you who is staying with us or if we've seen your son. What I can tell you is that they all come back here at 4:00 p.m. for the evening. Many of them hang out at that park over there during the day."

She faced me, looking straight in my eyes to make her point clear.

"Honey, do you understand what I'm telling you? They

line up here around 4:00 p.m. for the evening and many hang out at that park."

Looking at me intently, she repeated, "You *do* understand what I'm telling you?"

I did! She was another angel, making sure I didn't miss a beat with her message or the chance to find Nicky.

Thanking her, I quickly got in the car to search for Nicky at the park, but we didn't find him. A whole bunch of men were sitting around smoking and talking, but Nicky wasn't with them. He wasn't at the repair shop either. Anything can happen on the street. He was vulnerable, and we were on borrowed time.

Driving along farther down the road, I prayed intently as I scanned the area. Within a few minutes, I saw a tall, thin white guy dressed in pants hanging below his waistline and a hooded sweatshirt, which thankfully wasn't covering his face. Still, that couldn't be Nicky—he wasn't that thin, and this certainly wasn't what he was wearing a month earlier!

But on closer look, it *was* Nicky. Walking on the side of the road, looking like someone I would not want him to run into. He walked across the bridge as we were about to drive up alongside him. We waited to call out to him, not knowing what condition he was in or what he would do if startled. Crossing over the bridge, we made our move.

I rolled down the passenger-side window, so as not to startle him, and called out.

"Hey, good looking, do you need a ride?"

Nicky looked up and over at me with a smile of amazement.

"Mom, what are you doing here?"

"Looking for you."

"How long have you been looking?"

"Long enough to find you."

"Mom, I kept looking for your car, thinking I would see it. I just knew you'd find me! Who called you? How *did* you find me? Who helped you?"

"I believe God had something to do with it!"

Jumping out of the car, I ran over and hugged him, and he hugged me back.

"How about we go and get something to eat?"

"Okay, Mom. That sounds great. I'm starving. First we need to get my things at the Salvation Army."

Heading back to the Salvation Army to gather what few belongings he had, thanking them and saying good-bye, we then went to the repair shop. His car wasn't worth a dime. I paid for the towing service, and we signed the title over to them. The shop owner had a few words of wisdom to share as we were leaving.

"Nicholas, you mentioned some guy was going to buy your car, and you were going to buy the Mustang out front? Who was going to buy your car?"

"My friend that I met."

"What friend that you met?"

"My friend that I met at the Salvation Army who was living there."

"Son, you all pay about $5 a night there to live because you're homeless. How in the world would this guy have money to buy your broken-down car? And how in the world could you buy that Mustang sitting out there that costs $4,000 when you can't afford to pay for the towing expenses of your own car?"

Nicky nodded his head in agreement, knowing his thinking wasn't realistic.

"Nicholas, you have a mother who loves you an awful lot. She is here to help you. Go home and listen to her. She will do you right. You know that. Living out here on the street is not a good idea. Go home and get your life situated with her help."

I walked over to the other side of the counter where he was sitting and hugged him, thanking him for being an angel. We left to get a bite to eat before tackling the six-hour drive home.

Heading into the restaurant we were stopped in the parking lot by a young woman asking for money. She was crying, holding her hand out for anything she could get. I reached into my purse, gave her a few dollars, telling her to buy food, and we would pray for her. With tears flowing down her face, she thanked me.

As we entered the restaurant, the staff reprimanded me for the handout.

They had their reasons. I had mine.

As we waited for our food, Nicky began to tell us about the last three weeks, living on the street, and how he was starving and knew he had lost a lot of weight. He told us how his car had broken down and how he was determined to get himself out of his own mess, since he had gotten himself into the mess. The police questioned him on the street, and he made sure he was respectful to them. He couldn't sleep on benches at night, so he had to find other places to sleep that were well-lit. He was afraid he would be robbed, of who knows what. Nicky did hold a sign on the side of the street with another guy. Nicky was later told by the other housemates at the Salvation Army to stay away from that white guy, as he was on drugs and was bad news. They recognized, and were trying to protect him from, his own naïve thinking.

Nicky was also finding out the bad side of the digital world was even worse and was about to catch up to him. He had gone through three phones paying upgrade fees. He'd also been scammed by internet crooks who promised to loan him $30,000 if he sent them his bank account number, so he had sent them an image of his bank card. Nicky admitted there would be a sizable debt due to the phone purchases, upgrades, and bank scam that he would need help clearing up. He had been victimized, but was thankfully alive.

The Salvation Army had fed him and let him shower. They had played ping pong, and that evening there was supposed to be a ping pong match Nicky was sure he would win. He explained to the others that while growing up, his family had competitive ping pong matches. He also had attended prayer services at the Salvation Army, which was where he had prayed I would come looking for him.

It was about 6:00 p.m., and we were all tired. Getting into the car for the long drive home, Nicky stretched out in the back seat, about to fall asleep when my phone rang.

It was the detective who had been assigned to Nicky's case. I was surprised he was calling far sooner than I had been told to expect.

"Hello?"

"This is Detective O'Brian. I'm calling to speak to a Melissa Jacobus."

"This is she."

"I have been assigned to the case to try to find your son. I need to ask you a few questions."

"Not to interrupt you, but my son is with me. I'm driving back from Tuscaloosa, Alabama, where I found him."

"Excuse me . . . did you say he is with you in the car?"

"Yes, he is safe and in the car."

"Do you think you could drive by the police station on your way home so I can do a check on him?"

"Well, it's going to be pretty late when we get back to Atlanta, and no, I won't be making my way over there. You are welcome to come meet us at my house when we arrive around 11:00 p.m. tonight."

"No, I won't be able to do that. Will you put your son on the phone so I can talk to him to make sure he's fine?"

"Yes, here he is."

I handed the phone to Nicky and listened as he

answered the detective's questions. Then Nicky handed the phone back, saying the detective needed to talk to me again.

"Your son sounds like he's doing well. Will you please call your local police department tomorrow and have them do the welfare check so we can close the case?"

"Yes, I'll take care of it. Thanks for your help, and if you need anything else, you have my number."

"Could I ask you one more question before we hang up?

"Yes, what is it?"

"How did you find him? With the limited information you gave to the officer in filing the BOLO, how in the world did you find him? You didn't have much to go on."

"No, it wasn't, but it's all I had, along with lots of praying."

"I understand, but really, how did you find him? It would be impossible with the little information that you had to go on. How did you do it?"

Pausing, with a lump in my throat and tears in my eyes, but with complete confidence, I answered him.

"It was by the grace of God."

And with that, we hung up the phone and continued our faith-driven ride home.

The End

Actually, this is not the end, but a continued call for action that FASD is noted as a developmental disability, so those impacted can receive the services they need to begin living their lives the way God intended—happy, fulfilled, and understood.

Epilogue

Society's ignorance is "the accomplice" to the lack of awareness and training needed to understand and mitigate FASD, which perpetuates what could be prevented—homelessness and potential criminal behavior. When society replaces ignorance with knowledge, those with FASD will be able to celebrate their gifts, strengths, and well-deserved accomplishments, and lead happy, healthy lives.

Nicky was found, thank God. But I never thought he would be homeless and I'd have to go searching for him. He had been surrounded by the environmental prescription of protective factors, the social fabric of community support, an understanding employer, and a family that loved him and understood his FASD challenges—until he left home. Because FASD isn't recognized as a developmental disability, Nicky didn't have the clinical support and state services he needed to manage his challenges with FASD. Neither did Natalia. And neither did Maurice. FASD doesn't discriminate.

It's my prayer and life's mission to educate society about the FASD pandemic, to support those impacted by FASD, and to continue to "Be On the Lookout" for every Maurice, Natalia, and Nicky.

About the Author

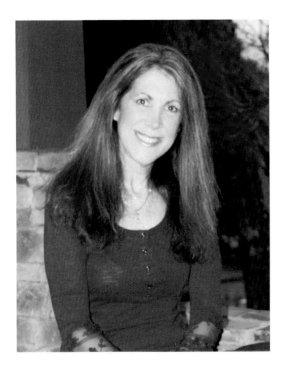

Melissa Jacobus has been advocating for her adopted children and the rights of all individuals with FASD since 1998. At the national level, she is a parent advocate and member of the Justice Task Force for the National Organization on Fetal Alcohol Syndrome (NOFAS), serves on the Advisory Committee for FASD Communities, and served as a member of the Speakers Bureau for the Centers for Disease Control's Fetal Alcohol Spectrum Disorders Southeast

Regional Training Center. In 2019, Ms. Jacobus was inducted into NOFAS' Tom and Linda Daschle FASD Hall of Fame.

Melissa is also active at the state level in Georgia. Among her accomplishments, in 2012, she presented at the Georgia Department of Behavioral Health and Developmental Disabilities Suicide Prevention Program and the Supreme Court of Georgia's Committee on Justice for Children. In 2013, her work led Governor Deal to designate September 9 as FASD Awareness Day, which has continued under the current governor, Brian Kemp. Melissa co-led the 2018 Atlanta Training on FASD at the State Bar of Georgia.

Melissa received a bachelor of science in broadcasting from the University of Florida. She worked for the Tribune Broadcasting Company and was awarded the company's highest honor for customer service before resigning in 1997 to devote herself full time to raising awareness and understanding of FASD. She lives in Atlanta, Georgia.

For more information on FASD, please visit the following:

National Organization on Fetal Alcohol Syndrome (NOFAS)

www.nofas.org

CDC Fetal Alcohol Spectrum Disorders (FASDs)

www.cdc.gov/ncbddd/fasd/index.html

American Academy of Pediatrics (AAP)

www.aap.org

www.aap.org/en-us/advocacy-and-policy/aap-health-initiatives/fetal-alcohol-spectrum-disorders-toolkit/Pages/default.aspx

www.healthychildren.org/English/health-issues/conditions/chronic/Pages/Fetal-Alcohol-Spectrum-Disorders.aspx

American College of Obstetricians and Gynecologists (ACOG)

www.acog.org

www.acog.org/en/Programs/FASD

Indian Health Service (IHS)

www.ihs.gov

www.ihs.gov/dccs/mch/fasd

University of Washington, Addictions, Drug and Alcohol Institute

www.depts.washington.edu/fadu/resources

Families Affected by Fetal Alcohol Spectrum Disorder (FAFASD)

www.fafasd.org

Double ARC Center for FASD

www.doublearc.org

Proof Alliance

www.proofalliance.org

FASD Communities

www.fasdcommunities.org

The Centre for Addiction and Mental Health (CAMH) Fetal Alcohol Spectrum Disorders (FASD)

www.camh.ca

www.camh.ca/en/health-info/mental-illness-and-addiction-index/fetal-alcohol-spectrum-disorder

The Canada Fetal Alcohol Spectrum Disorder Research Network (CanFASD)

www.canfasd.ca

www.canfasd.ca/topics/basic-information/

FASD Hub Australia - FASD Hub

www.fasdhub.org.au

www.fasdhub.org.au/fasd-information/understanding-fasd/